Study Guide for

Bowden and Greenberg's Children and Their Families: A Continuum of Care, Second Edition

WY159
Bow

Wolters Kluwer | Lippincott Williams & Wilkins
Health

Philadelphia · Baltimore · New York · London
Buenos Aires · Hong Kong · Sydney · Tokyo

Acquisitions Editor: Jean Rodenberger
Product Manager: Eric Van Osten
Editorial Assistant: Victoria White
Design Coordinator: Brett MacNaughton
Senior Designer: Joan Wendt
Manufacturing Coordinator: Karin Duffield
Prepress Vendor: Cadmus Communications, a Cenveo Company

9 8 7 6 5 4 3 2 1

Printed in China

ISBN-13: 9780781789660

Care has been taken to confirm the accuracy of the information presented and to describe generally accepted practices. However, the author, editors, and publisher are not responsible for errors or omissions or for any consequences from application of the information in this book and make no warranty, expressed or implied, with respect to the currency, completeness, or accuracy of the contents of the publication. Application of this information in a particular situation remains the professional responsibility of the practitioner; the clinical treatments described and recommended may not be considered absolute and universal recommendations.

The author, editors, and publisher have exerted every effort to ensure that drug selection and dosage set forth in this text are in accordance with the current recommendations and practice at the time of publication. However, in view of ongoing research, changes in government regulations, and the constant flow of information relating to drug therapy and drug reactions, the reader is urged to check the package insert for each drug for any change in indications and dosage and for added warnings and precautions. This is particularly important when the recommended agent is a new or infrequently employed drug.

Some drugs and medical devices presented in this publication have Food and Drug Administration (FDA) clearance for limited use in restricted research settings. It is the responsibility of the health care provider to ascertain the FDA status of each drug or device planned for use in his or her clinical practice.

LWW.COM

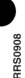

RRS0908

Preface

This Study Guide was developed by the instructional design firm of LearningMate and was reviewed by Marilee LeBon, Wendy Bowles, Kay Vorholt, Kim Joo, Angie Berger, and Mary Ann Foley to accompany the second edition of *Children and Their Families: The Continuum of Care* by Vicky R. Bowden, RN, DNSc and Cindy Smith Greenberg, DNSc, RN, CPNP. The study guide is designed to help you practice and retain the knowledge you've gained from the textbook, and it is structured to integrate that knowledge and give you a basis for applying it in your nursing practice. The following types of exercises are provided in each chapter of the study guide:

ASSESSING YOUR UNDERSTANDING

The first section of each study guide chapter concentrates on the basic information of the textbook chapter and helps you to remember key concepts, vocabulary, and principles.

- *Fill in the Blanks*
  Fill-in-the-blank exercises test important chapter information, encouraging you to recall key points.
- *Matching*
  Matching questions test your knowledge of the definition of key terms.
- *Sequencing*
  Sequencing exercises ask you to remember particular sequences or orders in, for example, testing processes and prioritizing nursing actions.
- *Short Answers*
  Short-answer questions cover facts, concepts, procedures, and principles of the chapter. These questions ask you to recall information as well as demonstrate your comprehension of the information.

APPLYING YOUR KNOWLEDGE

The second section of each study guide chapter consists of case study-based exercises that ask you to begin to apply the knowledge you've gained from the textbook chapter and that was reinforced in the first section of the study guide chapter. A case study scenario based on the chapter's content is presented, and then you are asked to answer some questions, in writing, related to the case study. The questions cover the following areas:

- Assessment
- Planning nursing care
- Communication
- Reflection

PRACTICING FOR NCLEX

The third and final section of the study guide chapters helps you practice NCLEX-style questions while further reinforcing the knowledge you have been gaining and testing yourself for throughout the textbook chapter and the first two sections of the study guide chapter. In keeping with NCLEX, the questions presented are multiple choice and scenario based, and ask you to reflect, consider, and apply what you know, and to choose the best answer from those offered.

ANSWER KEYS

The answers for all the exercises and questions in the study guide are provided at the back of the book, so you can assess your own learning as you complete each chapter.

We hope you find this study guide to be helpful and enjoyable, and we wish you every success in your studies toward becoming a nurse.

—*The Publishers*

Contents

The Child Developing within the Family

Learning Objectives

- Select strategies to integrate elements of family-centered care into patient care practices.
- Discuss selected family theories, describing their strengths, limitations, and application to nursing practice.
- Explain the family life cycle model as a framework for viewing family development across the life span.
- Describe different family structures.
- Describe the functions and roles of family members within the family.
- Examine the impact of selected family issues on the family system.
- Examine the cultural and religious influences that can affect child healthcare.

SECTION I: ASSESSING YOUR UNDERSTANDING

Activity A *Fill in the blanks.*

1. _____ _____ _____ is a philosophy of care that permeates all interactions between families and healthcare providers and places a high value on the contributions made by the family in relation to their healthcare needs.

2. _____ refers to two or more individuals who depend on one another for emotional, physical, and economic support.

3. The _____ function of the family provides for the continuation of society as well as the family.

4. The _____ function of the family provides for the emotional support of its members through love, encouragement, intimacy, and acceptance.

5. The _____ _____ is a high-quality, cost-effective approach to providing healthcare services that are accessible, continuous, comprehensive, family centered, coordinated, compassionate, and culturally effective.

6. A _____ is a disruption of psychological homeostasis, which occurs when a person faces an obstacle to important life goals that is, for a time, insurmountable through the utilization of customary methods of problem solving.

7. The _____ family, once considered the traditional family in many industrial societies, consists of a married couple and their immediate biologic children.

Activity B *Match the family theory in column A with its basic tenet listed in column B.*

Column A	Column B
____ 1. Family systems	a. The family is a unit that changes over time as a result of the physical and psychosocial transitions of
____ 2. Developmental	
____ 3. Family stress and coping	

____ **4.** Structural–
functional

____ **5.** Interactional

both adult and child members.

b. Focus is on the relationships between family members and how well the family performs its functions.

c. The family is a goal-directed unit made up of interdependent, interacting parts that endure over a period of time.

d. Focus is on the way in which family members relate to one another

e. Evaluates the impact of acute, unanticipated, and severe external events on the family system.

Activity C *Briefly answer the following.*

1. Define the term *family* using three different definitions used in family-centered practice.

_____

_____

_____

2. Describe the developmental issues that may occur when a couple decides to divorce.

_____

_____

_____

3. Give two definitions of family-centered care.

_____

_____

_____

4. List two issues that couples may encounter when attempting an international adoption.

_____

_____

_____

5. Describe three strategies that nurses may use to support children and their adoptive families.

_____

_____

_____

6. List three interventions nurses can use to enhance family-centered care for their patients.

_____

_____

_____

Activity D *Match the definitions in column A with the terms listed in column B.*

Column A

____ **1.** A source of stress that can cause tension for an individual or family

____ **2.** Values, beliefs, norms, and life ways of a particular group that guide their thinking, decisions, and actions in patterned ways

____ **3.** Organized system of commonly held beliefs, rituals, and observances in the worship of God or gods

____ **4.** Location of the family member in the family structure

____ **5.** How the family is organized

____ **6.** Biophysiologic characteristics of a population group that make it different from others

Column B

a. Culture

b. Religion

c. Demand

d. Race

e. Position

f. Structure

SECTION II: APPLYING YOUR KNOWLEDGE

Activity E *Consider this scenario and answer the questions.*

A nurse is performing a physical assessment on 16-year-old Chad who is brought to the emergency room with head trauma after a bike accident. The physician tells the nurse that Chad may need surgery to reduce the swelling in his brain. The only person available to give consent is Melinda, a friend of the family, who has a son Chad's age. Melinda states that her son and Chad have been "like brothers" growing up together in the neighborhood. Chad has been living with Melinda and her family since his mother's death in a car accident 3 months ago. Melinda does not yet have legal guardianship over Chase and there is no one else listed as "next of kin." Chase tells the nurse that Melinda is "all he has left now" and he doesn't know what he would do without her.

1. Based on the definitions of family, what is Melinda's relationship with Chad?

   _____

   _____

   _____

2. What nursing services would the nurse provide for this family based on the philosophy of family-centered care?

   _____

   _____

   _____

SECTION III: PRACTICING FOR NCLEX

Activity F *Choose the best answer.*

1. The nurse watches as a family comes together in support of a 13-year-old member diagnosed with leukemia. What function of the family is portrayed in this scenario?
   a. Affective
   b. Reproductive
   c. Economic
   d. Socialization

2. The pediatric nurse provides care to patients and their families in relation to optimizing the growth and development of the child. Which of the following encompasses this tenet?
   a. The child is a separate entity within the family.
   b. The focus of pediatric nursing is on the family.
   c. The philosophy of pediatric care is called *child-centered care*.
   d. The child cannot be viewed apart from the family who molded him or her

3. The nurse practicing family-centered care in a pediatric clinic recognizes that there are factors that make actualizing this type of care problematic. One of these factors is
   a. An increase in services
   b. Increase in family role stress
   c. An increase in staffing
   d. A decrease in cultural diversity

4. The parents of a family of five encourage their children to further their education by attending college. The family function involved in this action is
   a. Affective
   b. Healthcare
   c. Socialization
   d. Economic

5. A nurse attempts to define the word *family* to a student nurse. Which of the following is the description provided by the U.S. Census?
   a. Whomever the patient says it is
   b. Group of two or more persons related by blood, marriage, or adoption who are residing together
   c. Two or more persons who are related in any way—biologically, legally, or emotionally
   d. Two or more individuals who depend on one another for emotional, physical, and economic support

6. The nurse caring for children and their families knows that the basis for family-centered health care is
   a. The premise that a positive adjustment to a child's level of health and development

requires the involvement of the whole family

b. The technology that allows healthcare providers to care find cures and new treatment for disease states

c. The nurse is the individual ultimately responsible for the healthcare of the child

d. The interdisciplinary healthcare team involved in the care of the child and family

7. Which of the following activities best reflects the philosophy of practicing family-centered care?

a. A nurse strictly enforces the visiting hours to enhance security on the unit.

b. A nurse plans individual playtime for patients to give the parents a break from child care.

c. A nurse encourages family visiting in the postanesthesia room

d. A nurse reports to the parents the child care decisions made at interdisciplinary conferences.

8. A nurse recommends a medical home for a patient who has Down syndrome. Which of the following statements best describes the concept of a medical home?

a. The medical home refers to the house or hospital providing care.

b. The medical home refers to a specific healthcare team providing care.

c. The medical home provides high-quality, cost-effective healthcare services

d. The medical home provides free healthcare services to the needy.

9. The nurse caring for children and their families views the family as a goal-directed unit made up of interdependent interacting and enduring parts. This is an example of which of the following family theories?

a. Family systems approach

b. Developmental approach

c. Family stress and coping theory

d. Structural–functional theory

10. A family nurse interviews a couple with two children ages 13 and 15. The couple asks for guidance in setting limits for their children.

What is the nurse's best response in this situation?

a. "The rules you set for your family should remain the same from childhood to the adolescent years."

b. "Adolescents need stricter rules to keep them safe in their changing environment."

c. "Family rules should be adapted as your adolescents seek more independence."

d. "Family rules are dictated by the demands of society on the family and how the family responds to stressors."

Activity G *Choose all answers that apply.*

1. The nurse working in a family healthcare clinic attempts to provide family-centered care to all patients. Which of the following are key elements of this care?

a. Incorporating into policy the recognition that the healthcare service system is the constant in a child's life

b. Recognizing that the family is at the center of the healthcare plan

c. Facilitating family/professional collaboration at all levels of hospital, home, and community care

d. Exchanging information regarding the care plan to families and professionals on a need-to-know basis

e. Treating all patients the same regardless of their ethnic, racial, spiritual, social, economic, educational, and geographic diversity

f. Encouraging and facilitating family-to-family support and networking

2. The nurse providing family-centered care in a hospital setting is aware of the tenets of the family system approach that state that

a. The functional goal of the family system is to ensure survival, continuity, and growth of its components

b. The closed system depends on the interactions with the surrounding environment to achieve growth and change

c. As a unit, the family has boundaries that separate it from other systems

d. The family unit belongs to the many other systems that impinge on its boundaries

e. The family that has much exchange with the environment is one that resists change

f. A closed unit family depends on edict and law and order, and operates through force, both physical and psychological

3. A nurse caring for patients and their families in a community healthcare clinic uses Duvall's theory of family life cycles. These cycles are divided into eight stages based on

a. Major change in family size

b. Change in position of power in the family

c. Developmental stage of the youngest child

d. Work status of the primary wage earner

e. Number of children in the family

f. Number of adults in the family

Activity H *Fill in the blanks.*

1. The nurse caring for families in a community setting is aware that a _____ _____ can be defined as any group of adults (with or without children) most of whom are unrelated by blood or marriage, who live together, primarily for the sake of some ideologic goal for which a collective household is deemed essential.

2. The nurse counselor knows that the _____ determines the role that each family member should play to carry out the functions of the family.

Advocating for Children and their Families

- Review various factors and issues in the socio-political and medical arenas that affect the care of children and their families.
- Describe selected strategies that nurses, parents, and the community can use to promote health maintenance in children.
- Describe ethical principles that may affect the care of children and their families in either standard clinical or research settings.
- Review and contrast the legal rights of children, emancipated minors, and parents.
- List safety and documentation strategies unique to caring for children who are involved in research studies.
- Identify public, private programs and community sources of public healthcare and support for children and their families.
- State the educational programs available to support children with special healthcare and learning needs.

SECTION I: ASSESSING YOUR UNDERSTANDING

Activity A *Fill in the blanks.*

1. A nurse who acts to safeguard and to advance the interests of other persons as a means to help meet their healthcare needs is acting as a child _____.

2. The nurse who attempts to improve access to needed care and reduces gaps or duplication in services by developing and implementing an appropriate plan of care is acting as a care coordinator or _____ _____.

3. The nurse must be sensitive to patient confidentiality and must be aware of the _____ _____ _____ _____ _____ guidelines, which protect patients' privacy in healthcare settings, including hospitals, doctors' offices, and clinics.

4. To ensure the most comprehensive array of resources for their members, communities should undertake periodic _____ _____ to identify service demands that are not being met.

5. The _____ _____ _____, required by the Joint Commission, is formed to educate healthcare professionals, patients, and families about ethical issues and to provide individual case consultation and recommendations based on an ethical analysis of the relevant facts and feelings of all parties.

6. _____ _____ is a legal condition whereby a person can be said to have given consent based upon an appreciation and understanding of the facts and implications of an action.

Activity B *Match the terms in column A with the proper definition listed in column B.*

Column A

____ **1.** Sanctity of life

____ **2.** Beneficence

____ **3.** Assent

____ **4.** DNR/DNAR order

____ **5.** Innovative therapy

____ **6.** Quality of life

____ **7.** Informed consent

____ **8.** Justice

____ **9.** Emancipation

Column B

a. Acceptable state of life

b. Self-determination for medical care after consultation with physician

c. Agreement to participate in procedure or research

d. A respect for life being sacred

e. New and unproved interventions to gather new information

f. Doing good and avoiding harm

g. Decision not to attempt cardiopulmonary resuscitation

h. Process by which an individual becomes liberated from authority figures

i. Distribution of burden and benefits among the population of interest

Activity C *Briefly answer the following.*

1. Identify three strategies that nurses can use when caring for children and their families to improve child health.

_____

_____

_____

2. List three opportunities that are available to nurses to enable them to work in the community and support community health needs.

_____

_____

_____

3. Briefly define the role of the parents in advocating for their child's healthcare.

_____

_____

_____

4. Describe the role of the community in improving the health of children and families.

_____

_____

_____

5. List four services that communities could offer to support children and their families.

_____

_____

_____

6. Briefly describe the goals of the Head Start program.

_____

_____

_____

SECTION II: APPLYING YOUR KNOWLEDGE

Activity D *Consider this scenario and answer the questions.*

Rupa is a 37-year-old single mother of two children: a healthy 7-year-old boy, Devraj, and a 5-year-old girl, Ela, who was diagnosed with cerebral palsy (CP) shortly after birth. Ela exhibits signs of the spastic type of CP, including muscle contractures, spastic weakness, and difficulty with fine and gross motor skills. She also has average intelligence with minor hearing and speech deficits.

Rupa brings Ela to the health clinic for a physical required for entrance to kindergarten in the fall. During the focused health history, she confides to the nurse that she is worried about finding care for Ela because her mother, who was caring for Ela while she was at work, is no longer available to do so because of health reasons. Rupa states that her sister who lives next door is filling in for her temporarily while on maternity leave, but will eventually be going back to work herself.

The nurse elicits general information regarding Ela's treatment to date and finds out that she has had selective dorsal rhizotomy (SDR), a neurosurgical procedure performed to reduce muscle stiffness and spasticity. She also visits a physical therapist to improve her motor function and ambulation, and a speech therapist on an outpatient basis.

1. What measures can the nurse take to effectively advocate for Ela and her family, and perform the key role of care coordinator/case manager?

   _____

   _____

2. What is the role of the family in accessing and delivering care to Ela?

   _____

   _____

3. How can the community help improve the health of children and families like Rupa's? What is the nurse's role in ensuring that community services exist and are easily accessible to the public?

   _____

   _____

SECTION III: PRACTICING FOR NCLEX

Activity E *Choose the best answer.*

1. The nurse working with children with psychosocial disorders uses the Internet to research national programs that aid children and families. Which of the following national programs that focuses on the nurses' role in the prevention and early identification of psychosocial morbidities and overweight would be most helpful to this nurse's cause?

   a. Children's Defense Fund

   b. Keep Your Child/Yourself Safe and Sound (KySS) program

   c. American Academy of Pediatrics' Bright Futures in Practice

   d. American Medical Association Guidelines for Adolescent Preventive Services

2. A child is placed in hospice for palliative care. Which of the following interventions would be appropriate for this child's care?

   a. Ventilator therapy

   b. Pain medication

   c. Dialysis

   d. Vasoactive medication

3. A nurse cares for a neonate with anencephaly whose parents ask her about the doctor's recommendation for a do not resuscitate (DNR) order. What would be the nurse's best response?

   a. "Withholding medical treatment with a DNR order will spare your baby pain by hastening death."

   b. "I understand your hesitation, but this order is in the best interest of your baby."

   c. "You should know that the presence of a DNR order means that basic care such as suctioning and oxygen administration will be discontinued."

   d. "I realize this is a difficult decision to make. Do you have any questions about the process?"

4. The pediatric nurse caring for newborns with severe disabilities reviews the federal regulations that discuss criteria for withholding medically beneficial treatment, which includes

   a. Unconsciousness

   b. Futile treatment

   c. Invasive medical interventions

   d. Irreversible brain damage

5. A nurse explains to the parents of a child with leukemia the risks and benefits of trying innovative treatment and tells them:

   a. "Innovative treatments are new, but are fully assessed for safety and efficacy."

   b. "Innovative treatments are entirely different methods of treating diseases."

   c. "Innovative treatments are performed with the intent of gathering new information."

   d. "Innovative therapies can be an extension of existing methods to new indications."

6. A 12-year-old with juvenile diabetes and her parents are considering participation in a research study. The nurse explains to them that informed consent stipulates what they should know about the study, including

   a. They will have access to the findings

   b. They can only ask questions prior to the research

   c. What they are agreeing on is part of standard care

   d. They will know who the investigator is and how to contact him

7. A nurse helping patients apply for Medicaid knows that the following individuals qualify for the program:

   a. All children in federally funded daycare or foster care, regardless of income level

   b. All pregnant women with family income at or below 100% of the federal poverty level

   c. All children born after September 30, 1993, with family income up to 100% of the federal poverty level

   d. All infants born to Medicaid-enrolled women for as long as the mother is enrolled

8. A nurse advocating for a low-income pregnant woman and her 2-year-old child considers the Maternal and Child Health Services Block Grant state program for assistance. The goals of this program include

   a. Providing access to maternal and child health services regardless of income

   b. Providing prenatal, delivery, and postpartum care to at-risk women

   c. Providing free immunizations for all school-aged children not previously immunized

   d. Providing rehabilitation services for all mentally disabled members of the community

9. The nurse researching studies for her patients is aware of the principles that govern the ethical conduct of research, and weighs the benefits and risks associated with a patient's participation in a study. This principle is called

   a. Confidentiality

   b. Justice

   c. Beneficence

   d. Respect

10. A nurse is caring for a pregnant woman who is at risk for nutritional problems resulting from her income level. An appropriate referral for this woman would be

    a. Women, Infants and Children (WIC)

    b. Medicaid

    c. Supplemental Security Income (SSI)

    d. American Disabilities Act

Activity F *Choose all answers that apply.*

1. Pediatric nurses need to be familiar with the key initiative known as Healthy People 2010: National Health Promotion and Disease Prevention Objectives for the Year 2010. Which of the following areas were identified by this initiative as needing improvement?

   a. Immunization rates

   b. Injury and violence prevention

   c. Identification of psychosocial morbidities

   d. Prevention of childhood illnesses

   e. Maternal, infant, and child care

   f. Physical activity and fitness

2. Nurses must be aware of the principles of informed consent when advocating for patients. Which of the following are principles of this legal condition?

   a. Adults have the right to self-determination for medical care after consultation with a physician or other healthcare provider.

   b. Children older than the age of 12 can legally give informed consent for procedures.

   c. Informed consent must be voluntary and based upon information about risks and benefits of treatment.

   d. Parents of minors must be cognitively and mentally competent to make decisions for their child's care.

   e. Parents have the sole right to decide whether their decision is in the child's best interest.

   f. The child has the sole right to dissent if the intervention is deemed essential to his or her welfare.

Activity G *Fill in the blanks.*

1. _____ is a form of health insurance for low-income, disabled, and elderly persons that focuses on primary acute and long-term care, and only reimburses for services.

2. _____ provides money to states, which determine how it will be used to improve the health of all women and children, especially those at high risk or living in poverty.

3. _____ _____ _____ _____ _____ is an assistance program developed in 1997 as a successor to the Aid to Families with Dependent Children (AFDC) program to provide cash assistance to indigent American families with dependent children.

Principles and Physiologic Basis of Growth and Development

- Explain 10 principles fundamental to understanding the growth and development processes of children.
- Examine the biologic and environmental factors that can influence the growth and developmental processes in children.
- Describe the development of the body systems in children from birth through adolescence.
- Articulate selected theories that describe the psychosocial, cognitive, interpersonal, sexual, and moral development of children from birth through adolescence.
- Choose strategies the nurse can use to institute the process of developmental surveillance.

SECTION I: ASSESSING YOUR UNDERSTANDING

Activity A *Fill in the blanks.*

1. _____ refers to changes in size and function of the whole body or any part of the body.

2. Limited early social, educational, and environmental experiences place the child at "risk" for _____ delays.

3. Alcohol, heroin, and thalidomide are environmental factors called _____, which affect growth and development.

4. _____ patterns of growth and development within a certain time frame describe normal or average development.

5. The process by which living things transmit genetic codes to their offspring is _____.

6. Environmental consequences of reinforcement or punishment is _____ conditioning.

7. The term *developmental* _____ is the active and intentional evaluation of the child and family to identify those who may be at risk for developmental variation.

8. _____ refers to development in a head-to-toe fashion.

9. The rhythmic beat of the heart has begun by the _____ week and can be heard with a stethoscope by the 16th week.

10. The _____ reflex protects the infant from ingesting food substances that the gastrointestinal system is too immature to digest.

11. _____ has a major impact on behavior and development, and influences the dynamic interactions between the child and other people in the environment, especially the parents.

Activity B *Match the theorists in column A with the examples listed in column B.*

Column A

_____ **1.** Bandera/Sears

_____ **2.** Maslow/Rogers/ Ellis

_____ **3.** Kohlberg

_____ **4.** Elkind

_____ **5.** Piaget

_____ **6.** Freud

_____ **7.** Gilligan

_____ **8.** Gardner

_____ **9.** Pavlov/Watson

_____ **10.** Erickson

Column B

a. A 16-year-old told his mom, "I have to have this haircut; everyone will be watching me."

b. Moral development in which females focus on issues and how interpersonal relationships will be affected

c. The 18-month-old child picks up the toy and places it in the toy box after observing his sibling placing toys in the toy box

d. Emphasis is on the here and now; experiences within the environment and family can either promote or hinder growth

e. Personality based on epigenetic principle with predetermined steps at maturational levels with stages resulting in negative or positive outcomes

f. Multiple intelligences, child excels in math, and the sibling has an exceptional talent for understanding literature

g. Sequential development occurs to attain higher levels; levels relate to rationale for the moral decisions

h. Cognitive development with stages to explain how assimilation and accommodation of information is accomplished; adult understanding achieved through sequences of development

i. Stages include oral, anal, phallic, latency, and genital, and provide direction in handling children's sexual and aggressive drives

j. The child learns behavior through conditioned responses, which is termed *classical conditioning*

Activity C *Write the correct sequence for cephalocaudal gross motor development in the boxes.*

1. Hand control

2. Leg and foot control

3. Head control

4. Arm control

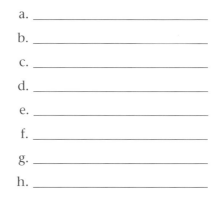

Activity D *Briefly answer the following.*

1. List factors that may cause malnutrition in the infant and child?

   a. _____

   b. _____

   c. _____

   d. _____

   e. _____

   f. _____

   g. _____

   h. _____

2. Define environmental factors and list four examples that affect growth and development.

   Environmental factors:_____

   _____

   _____

   a. _____

   b. _____

   c. _____

   d. _____

3. What are Kohlberg's six stages of moral reasoning? Briefly describe each stage.

   a. _____

   b. _____

   c. _____

   d. _____

   e. _____

   f. _____

4. What are the ages and expectations for the development of hearing?

   a. _____

   b. _____

   c. _____

   d. _____

5. What are the 10 principles necessary to understand the growth and development processes of children?

   a. _____

   b. _____

   c. _____

   d. _____

   e. _____

   f. _____

   g. _____

   h. _____

   i. _____

   j. _____

SECTION II: APPLYING YOUR KNOWLEDGE

Activity E *Consider the scenario and answer the questions.*

Emily is 2 years old and takes toys away from the other children. Her parents are embarrassed and concerned that Emily isn't learning to play with other children.

1. What cognitive stage of development does Emily's behavior demonstrate according to Piaget?

   _____

   _____

2. What explanation concerning Emily's behavior should be given to the parents by the nurse?

   _____

   _____

SECTION III: PRACTICING FOR NCLEX

Activity F *Answer the following questions.*

1. A child who is not walking by _____ months of age probably should be evaluated for developmental delays.
   a. 12 months
   b. 14 months
   c. 16 months
   d. 18 months

2. By _____ months of age, infants should be able to sit upright for long periods of time.
   a. 5
   b. 6
   c. 8
   d. 9

3. Identify the age at which children should be able to perform physical tasks of skipping, hopping, and walking down steps using alternating feet.
   a. 2 years
   b. 3 years
   c. 4 years
   d. 5 years

4. Which of the following best demonstrates how Maslow viewed human needs?
   a. Circular
   b. Hierarchical
   c. Triangular
   d. Continuum

5. Which of the following theories place importance on the experiences within the environment either reinforcing or eliminating the behaviors?
   a. Operant conditioning
   b. Cognitive social
   c. Social
   d. Psychosexual

6. A 5-year-old child at the clinic for a wellness checkup becomes upset after learning she is to receive an injection. Which of the following is the best nursing intervention by the nurse considering her growth and development?

   a. Give information about the medication and where it will be given.

   b. Explain that the hurting only lasts a few minutes and it will be quick.

   c. Ask the mom to step outside and have another nurse assist.

   d. Give the child a syringe, a simple explanation, and administer the injection.

7. Select the most appropriate toy for a hospitalized 9-month-old infant.

   a. A soft block for grasping and teething

   b. A push/pull toy to navigate in the bed

   c. A pillow to play peek-a-boo

   d. A container to place shapes through the openings

8. The mother reports that her 13-month-old child has been walking for 4 weeks, but walks like a duck and sometimes stumbles. Which of the following is accurate information to share with the parent concerning the child's locomotion?

   a. The walking should be more stable after 4 weeks of walking.

   b. Holding his hand as he walks should be done until he is more stable.

   c. If this continues for another 3 to 4 weeks, we will evaluate his walking.

   d. This is characteristic of a child who has been walking for this length of time.

9. Which of the following extremity positions would a term newborn assume?

   a. Outstretched arms and frog legs with flexed knees

   b. A flexed position similar to the position in utero

   c. Various positions by individual newborns

   d. The arms usually are flexed and legs extended

10. The nurse completes a newborn assessment and documents transient strabismus. Select the correct interpretation of this physical assessment characteristic.

    a. The newborn will need a referral to further evaluate her eyes.

    b. This is a very common occurrence among Asian populations.

    c. The condition is common at birth and should resolve in a few months.

    d. Eyes and ears develop at the same time, so both could be abnormal.

11. A 14-year-old has the need to have everything perfect—from her hair to her shoes—and spends an inordinate amount of time getting dressed, inconveniencing everyone in the family. Which of the following explains this behavior?

    a. Elkind called this *imaginary audience* and *personal fable* expected in adolescence.

    b. Piaget described this as accommodation to the adolescent's self-interest.

    c. This behavior as consistent with Maslow's identity versus role confusion stage.

    d. The example demonstrates Kohlberg's stage termed *interpersonal concordance.*

12. Which of the following screening tools is most appropriate and widely used for developmental assessments of children?

    a. Developmental journal

    b. Denver II Assessment Tool

    c. Numeric rating scale for growth and development

    d. Cognitive assessment scale

13. When caring for a 17-year-old undergoing surgery for a small laceration of the leg, which intervention by the nurse would be appropriate?

    a. Show a detailed visual of the surgery to parents and the adolescent.

    b. Allow the adolescent to "pretend" the repair procedure on a display.

    c. Give a pamphlet detailing the surgery, and preoperative and postoperative care.

    d. Explain the surgery, pre- and postoperative care, and allow an opportunity for questions.

14. The nurse caring for a 10-month-old uses talking and visual cues such as eye contact, smiling, and waving. Select the most accurate statement concerning visual cues.
    a. Talking to the infant is sufficient because of auditory sensitivity.
    b. Visual cues are an essential element of developing language skills.
    c. Verbal cues are more important for an infant who seldom uses visual cues.
    d. Infants are better at verbal than visual skills because hearing begins in utero.

15. The mother of 2-year-old twins reports to the nurse that the boy twin has fewer vocabulary words and verbalizes less than the girl twin. Select the explanation the nurse should give the mother.
    a. We will need to evaluate further because both are at the same developmental level.
    b. Girls in general are more advanced than boys in acquiring verbal language.
    c. Girls speak sooner than boys and, by age 3 years, the language skills will be the same.
    d. This could be a developmental delay and hearing should be tested for the boy twin.

16. The mother of an 18-month-old asks the nurse if her child will be as tall as her adult cousins. The infant currently weighs 26 lb and is 32 in tall. Calculate the expected height and weight that the infant will be as an adult to share with the mother.
    Answer: _____.

17. The healthcare provider is conducting preconceptual counseling for a couple who are of Ashkenazi Jewish heritage. Select the question that would be essential to ask the couple considering the common diseases affecting population groups?
    a. Have you been tested for the cystic fibrosis gene?
    b. Has any one in your family been born with a cleft lip and/or palate?
    c. Is there a family history of Tay-Sachs disease?
    d. Do you know if your family has had a child born with club feet?

18. A 4-year-old runs into the path of a car and is hospitalized. According to Fowler, which nursing intervention should be implemented to support faith development?
    a. Explain all facts, events, and procedures that are unfamiliar in the hospital setting.
    b. Allow the child to talk about his or her faith and list beliefs that are important.
    c. Offer prayer several times throughout the day for comfort and relaxation.
    d. Reinforce to the child that what happened is not because of being bad.

19. Select all of the following behaviors the nurse would expect to see in a 3-year-old in assessing growth and development.
    a. Walks stairs using alternating feet
    b. Chooses a finger food instead of soup
    c. Prefers being dressed by others
    d. Jumps rope with sibling
    e. Can identify gender
    f. Colors within a large border

CHAPTER 4

Infancy (Newborn–11 Months)

Learning Objectives

- Describe developmental milestones for neonates and infants, and state measures to enhance meeting these milestones.
- Discuss the needs of the infant related to hygiene, personal care, nutrition, elimination, and safety.
- Select age-appropriate interventions to promote healthy personal and social development of the infant.
- Select interventions to promote illness and injury prevention for the infant and the family.

SECTION I: ASSESSING YOUR UNDERSTANDING

Activity A *Match the term in column A with the proper definition in column B.*

Column A	Column B
____ **1.** Acid mantle	**a.** Gastrointestinal pain
____ **2.** Colostrum	**b.** Premilk
____ **3.** Kilocalorie	**c.** Protective secretions of sebaceous glands
____ **4.** Colic	**d.** First stool
____ **5.** Meconium	**e.** Energy content of food

Activity B *Fill in the blanks.*

1. The folds in the infant's _____ and perineal area are especially prone to rashes because they are warm and moist.

2. By the age of _____ months, the infant has developed enough motor control to coordinate both hands at once.

3. Infants commonly have a regular fussy period during the day, usually around _____ pm to midnight.

4. Most hospitals will not discharge an infant unless there is a _____ available to transport the child.

5. _____ is the process whereby the parent or other caregivers screen the child's environment for safety hazards and use measures to eliminate those hazards.

Activity C *Briefly answer the following.*

1. Describe the "REST" regimen for managing the child with colic.

_____

_____

_____

2. List three identifiable behaviors that indicate attachment is occurring between parent and child.

_____

_____

_____

3. How long can expressed breast milk and prepared commercial formula be safely kept in the refrigerator?

_____

_____

_____

4. Why should an infant never be fed by propping the bottle or by positioning it on a pillow or blanket to hold the bottle in the baby's mouth?

_____

_____

_____

SECTION II: APPLYING YOUR KNOWLEDGE

Activity D *Consider the scenario and answer the questions.*

A nurse is working on the mother/baby unit at the community hospital. One of the patients is an 18-year-old single mother who gave birth to her first child. The mother and baby are being discharged today. Upon entering the room, the nurse notices the mother looking frustrated and nervous as she is trying to change the infant's diaper while the child is crying loudly. The mother bursts into tears and exclaims, "I don't know what I am doing! How can I go home and take care of this baby by myself?"

1. How would the nurse intervene initially?

_____

_____

2. After assisting the mother with the diaper change, the infant is swaddled and place in her mother's arms. Immediately the child stops crying and calms down. What key questions and assessment areas would need to be addressed when developing this patient's discharge plan?

_____

_____

3. What would be the priorities in this patient's discharge plan?

_____

_____

SECTION III: PRACTICING FOR NCLEX

Activity E *Choose the best answer.*

1. The mother of a 2-week-old girl brings her baby into the pediatrician's office because the baby is only sleeping approximately 10 hours per day. The infant is alert, gaining weight, shows no signs of illness, and does not cry excessively. The mother insists there is something wrong because all the books she has read state that the average newborn should be sleeping more. What should the nurse say to the mother?

   a. "As you know, the average newborn sleeps 16 to 20 hours per day."
   b. "Your baby is healthy and may probably keep this pattern throughout his life."
   c. "Some young babies may even sleep as much as 23 hours per day."
   d. "Your baby is healthy and needs less sleep than average at this time."

2. The mother of a 3-month-old boy is preparing to return to work full-time. Their breast-feeding routine is well-established and the infant has never taken a bottle. The mother is trying to encourage the baby to take a bottle so he can drink expressed breast milk while the mother is away, but he refuses. The mother calls the nurse for advice. Which of the following should the nurse suggest to the mother?

   a. "Let someone else feed the baby the bottle; he may only refuse it from you."
   b. "Is it possible for you to delay your return to work for a little while?"
   c. "Keep trying; the baby will get hungry and will have to take a bottle."
   d. "Why don't you give the baby a commercial formula instead of breast milk?"

3. The pediatric nurse practitioner is trying to determine whether the infant is developing on schedule. Which of the following questions will most likely elicit more detailed information from the parents?

   a. "Is your son developing normally for a 9-month-old child?"
   b. "Is your son developing on schedule?"
   c. "Does your son smile when you smile or laugh?"
   d. "Describe the way your son moves about when you place him on the floor."

teaching the mother of a 4-day-
girl how to give her baby a bath.
of the following is the most important
ng instruction for this age?

a. "Gather all the supplies in advance to avoid leaving the baby unattended."

b. "Begin the bath by cleaning the baby's eyes from inner area to outer area."

c. "Do not submerge the baby in water until the dry cord falls off."

d. "Carefully check the water temperature. It should feel lukewarm to you."

5. The parents of a 4-month-old girl are taking their daughter to the beach for a vacation. They are concerned about protecting her from the sun and ask the nurse if it is okay to use sunscreen. Which of the following would be the best advice for the parents?

a. "Apply sunscreen sparingly, and use a hat and stroller canopy for the baby."

b. "Avoid the direct sun, and cover her with lightweight clothes, a hat, and sunglasses."

c. "You will need to keep her inside during the day. Take her out in the evening.

d. "Apply sunscreen sparingly, use sunglasses and a hat, and keep her in the shade."

6. The advance practice nurse practitioner has seen the same 11-month-old boy three times during the past 8 weeks for otitis media. His mother also mentions that he just saw a pediatric dentist for a cavity in a tooth that erupted 6 months ago. Which question would be most important for the nurse to ask?

a. "Is there a family history of ear infections?"

b. "Is there a family history of early tooth decay?"

c. "Is he going to bed with a bottle of milk or juice?"

d. "Does he have allergies or frequent colds?"

7. A nurse is caring for a 2-month-old boy. His mother is concerned that this infant is a thumb sucker and will not take a pacifier like his older brothers did. The mother asks the nurse how to make the baby accept the pacifier and not suck his thumb. How should the nurse respond?

a. "Your son will ultimately decide what he likes."

b. "Try to remove the thumb from his mouth."

c. "Try different types of one-piece pacifiers."

d. "You need to keep putting a pacifier in his mouth."

CHAPTER 5

Early Childhood (1–4 years)

Learning Objectives

- State the developmental surveillance and milestone concerns of children age 1 to 4.
- Discuss nutrition, elimination, hygiene, and personal care needs during the early childhood years.
- Select age-appropriate interventions to promote healthy personal and social development of children age 1 to 4.
- Select interventions to promote illness and injury prevention for the young child and the family.

SECTION I: ASSESSING YOUR UNDERSTANDING

Activity A *Match the terms in column A with the appropriate considerations from column B.*

Column A

____ **1.** Afternoon nap

____ **2.** Bathing

____ **3.** Bedtime

____ **4.** Mealtime

____ **5.** Teeth brushing

Column B

a. Child requires constant supervision

b. Child may start, but parents must finish

c. Not stressful, but not playtime

d. Finish at least 3 hours before bedtime

e. A routine is helpful

Activity B *Fill in the blanks.*

1. A good preschool should have the resources to identify any _____ disorders.

2. Giving a toddler a bath in the evening is not only good hygiene, but also a good _____ routine.

3. An active _____ and increased dream state account for most of the nightmares experience by toddlers.

4. Feeding and _____ are the first two areas in which the toddler will assert independence.

Activity C *Briefly answer the following.*

1. Describe the difference between night terrors and nightmares, including the proper parental reaction to each.

_____

_____

_____

2. Explain sibling rivalry and how parents should deal with it.

_____

_____

_____

3. What precautions should parents take to prevent their toddler from choking?

_____

_____

_____

APPLYING YOUR KNOWLEDGE

D *Consider the scenario and answer the questions.*

Janice Graves brings her 2½-year-old son, Devon, to the healthcare facility for a well-child checkup. During the visit, Janice says, "I'm so frustrated. I try to get Devon to eat different kinds of foods, but he all he ever seems to want to eat is macaroni and cheese. I don't know what to do." Janice also reports that Devon has temper tantrums. "I get so upset and scared because he holds his breath. I'm afraid to say no because he might throw a temper tantrum."

1. How might the nurse interpret Devon's desire to eat only macaroni and cheese?

   _____

   _____

2. What suggestions might the nurse give to promote Devon's nutritional intake?

   _____

   _____

3. How might the nurse respond to Janice's comments related to Devon's temper tantrums?

   _____

   _____

SECTION III: PRACTICING FOR NCLEX

Activity E *Choose the best answer.*

1. During a well-child visit, the mother of a 20-month-old girl asks the nurse if this is a good time to start toilet training her daughter. Which of the following comments would be most likely to lead to success?
   a. "Wait until she can describe the process of toileting."
   b. "There should be more than an hour between diaper changes."
   c. "She needs to be using five-word sentences."
   d. "Watch for signs such as an interest in imitating you."

2. The parents of a 30-month-old boy have just described a sleep disturbance the boy recently had. The nurse recognizes the event as a night terror. Which recommendation would be most appropriate?
   a. "Assure him it was only a bad dream."
   b. "Don't try to calm him or put him in bed."
   c. "Wait until morning to discuss the dream."
   d. "Don't let him watch TV before bedtime."

3. The parents of a 2-year-old boy are having trouble introducing new foods to the child and have asked the nurse for help. Which of the following comments provides the best advice?
   a. "Try serving the food in a different way."
   b. "Make him eat one bite to get dessert."
   c. "Show him how much you like the food."
   d. "Give him time out if he doesn't eat the food."

4. Which of the following suggestions would be most appropriate to give the parents of a 2½-year-old daughter about nutrition?
   a. "Allow the child to eat as many meals as she wants."
   b. "Give her the same foods that you are eating but about one quarter the amount."
   c. "Gradually increase her intake of foods containing fat."
   d. "Limit the amount of textures and tastes in the foods offered."

5. The nurse is observing a child in the clinic waiting room. The child is sitting on the chair next to his parent and is watching two other children playing. The child does not attempt to interact with them. The nurse interprets this as which type of play?
   a. Onlooker
   b. Solitary
   c. Parallel
   d. Associative

CHAPTER 6

Middle Childhood (5–10 years)

Learning Objectives

- State the developmental surveillance concerns and milestone accomplishments of middle childhood.
- Discuss the abilities of the school-aged child related to managing hygiene and personal care.
- Describe the nutritional requirements to promote optimum growth during middle childhood.
- Discuss the importance of engaging the child in physical activity with regard to developing lifelong health patterns of behavior.
- Select age-appropriate interventions to promote healthy personal and social development of the child.
- Describe strategies to help the child be successful in school.
- Select interventions to prevent illness and injury among children age 5 to 10 years and their families.

SECTION I: ASSESSING YOUR UNDERSTANDING

Activity A *Match the term in column A with the phrase in column B.*

Column A	Column B
____ 1. Fears	a. Special quality time
____ 2. Verbal bulling	b. Averting frustration
____ 3. Language	c. The neighbor's dog
____ 4. Sibling jealousy	d. Rudimentary skills
	e. Moves more gracefully
____ 5. Fine motor development	f. Influences personality
____ 6. Tantrums	g. Name calling, insults, threats
____ 7. Sports	h. Multiple commands
____ 8. Temperament	

Activity B *Match the term in column A with the phrase in column B.*

Column A	Column B
____ 1. Feeding strike	a. Gender identity as male or female
____ 2. Separation anxiety	b. Becoming upset when away from parental figures
____ 3. Hygiene	c. The order in which things happen or come
____ 4. Positive redirection	d. Activities that promote learning to read or write
____ 5. Sexuality	e. A period when certain foods are refused
____ 6. Early literacy	f. Verbally guiding child toward accepted behavior
____ 7. Sequencing	g. Conditions and practices that help to promote and preserve health
____ 8. Desensitization	h. When fear is conquered by approaching it little by little

Activity C *Place the following steps in the proper order.*

1. Dealing with a temper tantrum

    a. Call a time-out

    b. Exit the scene

    c. Express empathy

    d. Remain calm

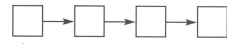

2. Exercise

    a. Warmup exercises

    b. Running around the track three times

    c. Eating a well-balanced breakfast

    d. Cool-down exercises

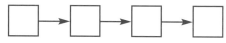

Activity D *Fill in the blanks.*

1. A ritualistic behavior common for this age is
   _____.

2. The preschooler's diet should be developed around the U.S. Department of Agriculture
   _____.

3. _____ has increasingly displaced activities such as reading and playing with friends.

4. Rowdy play should be avoided close to
   _____.

5. _____ play an important part in the child's development of self.

6. Children should be at least _____ years old before beginning organized sports.

7. _____ is a realistic, positive sense of self-worth and identity.

8. There is no formal statewide definition of _____ other than an age of eligibility requirement.

SECTION II: APPLYING YOUR KNOWLEDGE

Activity E *Briefly answer the following.*

1. Discuss how the nurse can assist the parents in dealing with a "difficult child."

   _____

   _____

   _____

2. Explain the most common mistake parents make in implementing time-outs, and outline the effective use of time-outs.

   _____

   _____

   _____

3. Why is play sometimes referred to as the *work* of the child?

   _____

   _____

   _____

4. Discuss the importance of peer relationships with this age group.

   _____

   _____

   _____

Activity F *Consider the scenario and answer the questions.*

   Easton, who is 5 years old, is being seen in the emergency room for fever, nausea, and vomiting. His mother and father are present. After the doctor sees Easton, he orders for medication to be given orally. As you approach Easton to give him the medication, he screams loudly and shouts, "No, no! I do not want to take that! Don't hurt me." Easton refuses to cooperate or take the medication.

1. Is Easton's behavior "normal" for his developmental age? Why or why not?

   _____

   _____

2. Describe a typical preschooler's reaction to hospitalization.

   _____

   _____

3. Develop a plan of care that addresses fears and concerns, and promotes self-esteem. Include a goal and interventions.

   _____

   _____

SECTION III: PRACTICING FOR NCLEX

Activity G *Choose the best answer.*

1. The nurse is caring for a 5-year-old boy. She is trying to determine whether he is achieving developmental milestones on schedule. Which of the following trigger questions will most likely elicit more detailed information from the parents?

   a. "Is your son developing normally for a 4-year-old?"

   b. "Do you think your son is developing on schedule?"

   c. "Can your son throw a ball?"

   d. "How does your son throw a ball?"

2. A 5-year-old girl will only eat peanut butter and jelly sandwiches and crackers. Her mother is frustrated and asks for guidance from the nurse. How should the nurse respond?

   a. "Feed her anything but peanut butter and jelly and crackers"

   b. "Continue to offer her other foods and this stage will pass."

   c. "Show her how much you like the new food you are offering."

   d. "Insist she take at least one bite of everything on her plate."

3. The father of a 7-year-old boy discusses with you that his son cannot seem to get into a good study pattern because of after-school activities, dinnertime, and then family time. What should the nurse recommend to the father?

   a. "Do not worry; these habits will develop over time."

   b. "Stop all after-school activities and focus on homework."

   c. "Encourage a routine and find a quiet place without distractions."

   d. "Remove all items from the room that the child enjoys to increase attention."

4. The mother of a 5-year-old boy is preparing to rejoin the workforce 3 days a week. She has enrolled her son in a preschool with an afternoon extended care program. The mother asks the nurse the best way to ensure a smooth transition into daycare. Which of the following is the most important recommendation?

   a. "Spend a few minutes at the center reading a book with your child."

   b. "Develop a morning routine, prepare the night before, and avoid rushing out the door."

   c. "Stay with your son during the first group activity to ease the transition."

   d. "Keep your goodbyes short; do not appear unsure about leaving."

5. The advance practice pediatric nurse practitioner is caring for a 5-year-old girl. The nurse practitioner is trying to determine whether the girl is achieving developmental milestones on schedule. Which of the following responses indicates that further evaluation is warranted?

   a. "My daughter holds her pencil in a fist."

   b. "My daughter can skip."

   c. "My daughter can walk on a balance beam."

   d. "My daughter knows her phone number and address."

6. The nurse is caring for 6-year-old twins. She is reviewing their diet and eating habits with their mother as part of a routine wellness examination. Which of the following responses indicates a need for further teaching about promoting healthy eating habits?

   a. "Tim is a good eater and Jim is a picky eater."

   b. "Both Tim and Jim eat a lot of peanut butter and jelly."

   c. "The boys don't like soda."

   d. "Tim likes juice, but only has it twice a week."

7. During a well-child examination, the mother confides to the nurse that her youngest son always eats at a different time and always demands a different menu from the rest of the family. How should the nurse respond?

   a. "You need to stop feeding him at a different time."

   b. "Feed him the same food as the rest of the family."

   c. "There are a couple of changes that you need to make."

   d. "You need to quit pampering the child at mealtimes."

8. The nurse is caring for a 5-year-old boy. During a routine wellness examination, his mother expresses her concern about her son's development. She believes that he has some developmental delays because he cannot do many of the same things that his 4-year-old cousin can do. The nurse reassures the mother that thus far he seems to be within the range of normal, but the mother is insistent there must be something wrong because he is not doing everything like his cousin. How should the nurse respond?

   a. "You shouldn't compare your son with other children his age."

   b. "Every child, including your son, develops at a different time."

   c. "Why don't we schedule a Denver II Developmental Screening Test?"

   d. "Your son seems to be developing normally; let's wait until your next visit."

9. The nurse is caring for a 5-year-old girl with two teenage brothers. Recently, the girl has begun to resist going to bed at a regular bedtime. The girl wants to stay up with the rest of the family and has consequently become very crabby in the morning. The mother is unsure about what to do and asks the nurse for some guidance. Which of the following would be the best approach?

   a. Let the girl stay up with her brothers and fall asleep when she is tired

   b. Engage in fun games before bedtime to tire the girl out

   c. Insist the girl go to bed at her bedtime

   d. Reestablish a consistent, relaxing bedtime routine

10. The nurse is conducting a routine wellness examination of a 5-year-old girl. The mother tells the nurse that her daughter is exceptionally bright and most likely gifted. The mother shares that she is working with her daughter every day to help her learn to read before she starts kindergarten this year. How should the nurse respond?

    a. "Reading together, trips to the library, and making your own books are best for a bright 5-year-old like your daughter."

    b. "The only accurate way to measure giftedness is through standardized testing."

    c. "Try reading together; teaching her to read at age 5 is not developmentally appropriate."

    d. "Forcing her to learn how to read now might be counterproductive."

CHAPTER 7

Promoting Healthy Lifestyles: Adolescence (11–21 years)

- State the age-appropriate developmental milestones of the adolescent years.
- Distinguish components of developmental surveillance unique to the adolescent population.
- Discuss the concerns of the adolescent related to hygiene and personal care.
- Describe challenges to maintaining optimum nutrition in the adolescent years.
- Describe activities that promote physical fitness in adolescents.

SECTION I: ASSESSING YOUR UNDERSTANDING

Activity A *Match the description in column A with the appropriate answer in column B.*

Column A

_____ 1. All school-aged children

_____ 2. Puberty

_____ 3. Self-advocacy

_____ 4. 12-year-old boys

_____ 5. 11-year-old girls

_____ 6. Menarche

Column B

a. Have achieved 90% of adult height and 50% of adult weight

b. The first menstruation

c. The sequence of events by which a child becomes a young adult

d. Assist the adolescent in seeking out, evaluating, and using information to promote his or her own health

e. Have achieved 80% of adult height and 50% of adult weight

f. Experience acceleration of growth of long bones

Activity B *Match the type of developmental milestone in column A with the description of the milestone in column B.*

Column A

_____ 1. Sexual

_____ 2. Physical

_____ 3. Play

_____ 4. Cognitive

_____ 5. Moral

Column B

a. Death is irreversible, universal, personal, but distant

b. Laws recognized as changeable

c. Genital stage

d. Adult cardiovascular rhythms achieved by age 16

e. Thrill-seeking behaviors

Activity C *Place the following developmental milestones in the proper sequence.*

1. Catches tennis ball with one hand

2. Puts right or left foot forward on command

3. Walks a straight line

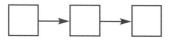

Activity D *Fill in the blanks.*

1. _____ is the sequence of events by which a child becomes a young adult.

2. _____ is considered the ultimate hallmark of late puberty for teenage girls.

3. _____ is a form of body art that is done with a third-degree burn to the skin and, after the burn heals, a design of scar tissue is left behind.

4. Adolescents are becoming more interested in _____ a type of plastic surgery to change the appearance of the body.

5. _____ is recommended for all female adolescents who are capable of becoming pregnant to reduce the risk of giving birth to a child with a neural tube defect.

6. The use of resistance methods to increase muscle ability to exert or resist force, known as _____, is popular among adolescents.

7. _____ is the most commonly used contraceptive among adolescents.

8. _____ is the most effective way to prevent sexually transmitted infections.

SECTION II: APPLYING YOUR KNOWLEDGE

Activity E *Briefly answer the following.*

1. Discuss dietary strategies for adolescents to ensure that they have a caloric intake of 1,500 to 2,400 calories per day.

   _____

   _____

   _____

2. Discuss the positive benefits of physical activity for the adolescent.

   _____

   _____

   _____

3. Initiation of sexual activity may begin during the latter school-aged years. Discuss the characteristics of an adolescent that engages in early sexual activity.

   _____

   _____

   _____

Activity F *Consider the scenario and answer the questions.*

   Ellie is 15 years old and is a freshman. Ellie is the second of four children and she is the oldest daughter in the family. Her parents are married and her immediate family lives in the area. She has always had a great deal of support from her family and friends. She has recently met a boy that is new to the area. He is from a single-parent home, he lives with his father, and they have recently been relocated to the area because of the father's job. Ellie has come to the office today for complaints of an earache. While there, her mother asks, without Ellie's knowledge, about preparing her daughter for sexual activity.

1. As the nurse, what should you discuss with the mother about teenage sexuality?

   _____

   _____

2. Ellie's mother asks you what characteristics she should look for that may be signs of early sexual activity, since Ellie has begun dating the boy that lives in a single-parent home.

_____

_____

3. Ellie's mother asks what are the most important things that she should discuss when talking to Ellie about sex.

_____

_____

SECTION III: PRACTICING FOR NCLEX

Activity G *Choose the best answer.*

1. The pediatric nurse is caring for an 11-year-old girl. She is trying to determine whether the girl is achieving developmental milestones on schedule. Which of the following trigger questions will most likely elicit more detailed information from the parents?
   a. "Is your daughter developing normally for an 11-year-old?"
   b. "Do you think your daughter is developing on schedule?"
   c. "Does your daughter like school?"
   d. "What does your daughter like best about school?"

2. A mother is attempting to provide a well-balanced diet for her 12-year-old daughter. The girl does not want to bring a "brown bag" lunch from home and prefers the lunches served in the cafeteria. The mother is concerned about the poor nutritional quality of the school lunches and asks for guidance from the nurse. How should the nurse respond?
   a. "Let her buy her lunch some days and take her lunch to school on others."
   b. "Let her prepare her own school lunches and avoid the cafeteria lunches."
   c. "She is old enough to make good food choices; it is up to her what she eats."
   d. "Let her prepare her own school lunches and then limit the number of days she buys."

3. The mother of a 13-year-old boy confides to the pediatric nurse practitioner that her son has recently had a nocturnal seminal emission. The mother is concerned and the nurse reviews "wet dreams" and the other male traits of puberty with the mother. Which of the following responses indicates a need for further discussion?
   a. "My son must be sexually active or having overly sexual thoughts to have a nocturnal emission."
   b. "My son's spontaneous erections and nocturnal emissions are very normal."
   c. "My son is not doing anything to cause the nocturnal emissions; they occur spontaneously."
   d. "My son is developing normally and the traits of puberty vary from child to child."

4. The pediatric nurse is caring for a 15-year-old boy who seems interested in making some of his own decisions regarding his care. The nurse knows that is important to promote this behavior. Why?
   a. It promotes self-advocacy and provides the adolescent with age-appropriate information.
   b. Adolescents report that they desire to receive healthcare from competent professionals and this actions shows this behavior.
   c. Healthcare providers should not allow these decisions if the child is still living at home and the parents are involved.
   d. Healthcare providers play an important role in helping to support adolescents during these challenging years.

5. Steven is being seen in the office for a case of folliculitis. He admits that he and some friends were at a shaving party. What statement indicates that he needs further education?
   a. "I understand that if I get a rash, I need to have it evaluated by a practitioner."
   b. "I do not understand how this happened. We rinsed the razors between uses."
   c. "The antibiotic cream helped to soothe the itching that I had."
   d. "I did not use Joey's razor. He is nasty and I did not want what he has."

6. The nurse is caring for a 14-year-old girl. She is reviewing diet and eating habits as part of a routine wellness examination. Which of the following would be the best question to assess daily fat intake?

   a. "Do you count the amount of fat in your diet?"

   b. "Can you tell me what you have eaten for the past 24 hours?"

   c. "How many fat grams do you eat in an average day?"

   d. "Do you eat any low-fat or fat-free foods?"

7. The nurse is caring for a 13-year-old girl. The nurse is assessing nutrition during a well-child examination. When the nurse reviews calcium intake, the girl indicates that she does not drink milk. How should the nurse respond?

   a. "Have you tried drinking chocolate milk?"

   b. "Can you tell me some other sources of calcium?"

   c. "Do you think you are getting enough calcium?"

   d. "What do you have on your cereal in the morning?"

8. Mandy is a 17-year-old that is being seen for complaints of being tired during the day and depressed mood. What is the best question that the nurse could ask to evaluate the patients sleep pattern?

   a. "Is there any family history if insomnia?"

   b. "How much sleep do you get at night?"

   c. "Discuss your sleep pattern for the past 2 weeks."

   d. "Do you sleep uninterrupted through the night?"

Health Assessment and Well-Child Care

Learning Objectives

- Describe the levels of prevention that are used as primary approaches to pediatric health teaching.
- List the childhood immunizations and their schedule of administration for those routine vaccines and identify the side effects associated with each of the vaccines.
- Discuss key components in the health assessment of children from infancy through adolescence and what is covered in each component (e.g., past medical history, social history, anticipatory guidance).
- Elicit a pediatric health history pertinent to either the health supervision needs or illness-related problems of children from birth through adolescence.
- Discuss key approaches to interviewing the child and the family based on developmental considerations, psychosocial/emotional considerations, and level of acuity of illness.
- Perform a basic physical examination on a child that reflects knowledge of the developmental differences in the various body systems from birth through adolescence.
- Identify how the physical examination process may need to be altered based on developmental considerations.
- Differentiate normal from abnormal findings obtained while either taking historical information or performing the physical examination.
- Discuss the healthcare areas that are covered during health surveillance visits of children of each age group.

- Select age-appropriate teaching techniques to relay anticipatory guidance and disease prevention information.

SECTION I: ASSESSING YOUR UNDERSTANDING

Activity A *Match the ausculatory site in column A with the description in column B.*

Column A

_____ 1. Aortic area

_____ 2. Pulmonic area

_____ 3. Erb's point

_____ 4. Tricuspid area

_____ 5. Mitral area

Column B

a. Second left intercostal space

b. Fifth right and left intercostals spaces

c. Second right intercostal space

d. Second and third intercostal spaces

e. Third to fourth intercostal space, lateral to left midclavicular line

Activity B *Match the deep tendon reflex in column A with the associated normal finding in column B.*

Column A

_____ 1. Achilles

_____ 2. Biceps

_____ 3. Quadriceps

Column B

a. Slight flexion of forearm

b. Partial extension of forearm

____ **4.** Brachioradialis

____ **5.** Triceps

c. Forearm flexion with palms turning upward

d. Partial extension of lower leg

e. Foot plantar flexion

Activity C *Fill in the blanks.*

1. A deviation called a _____ appears as a clef notch at the outer edge of the iris.

2. A history of severe _____ reaction to a vaccine or a vaccine's component is the only true contraindication to immunization.

3. What the adolescent and the parent say during an interview must be kept _____ from the other.

4. _____ is a large diffuse area of black and blue color caused by bleeding into the skin.

5. The _____ pulse rate is counted for 1 full minute.

SECTION II: APPLYING YOUR KNOWLEDGE

Activity D *Consider the scenario and answer the questions.*

    Jermaine and Claudia Persons bring their two sons, Michael, a 6-month old, and Jaron, a 4-year-old, to the clinic for a visit. The parents report that the children have been doing well. Michael demonstrates achievement of appropriate developmental milestones. Jaron is an active and talkative 4-year-old.

1. When assessing the Michael's reflexes, what would the nurse expect to find?

    _____

    _____

2. How would assessing anthropometric measurements for Michael differ from that for the 4-year-old?

    _____

    _____

3. Calculate the body mass index for Jaron who weighs 40 lb and is 42 in tall.

    _____

    _____

4. Would the nurse expect to administer any immunizations to either Michael or Jaron? If not, why not? If so, what immunizations would be appropriate?

    _____

    _____

SECTION III: PRACTICING FOR NCLEX

Activity E *Choose the best answer.*

1. When examining the eyes of an infant, which of the following would the nurse report as an abnormal finding?

    a. A cleft notch at the outer edge of the iris

    b. A bilateral blue tint to the sclera

    c. Intermittent crossed eyes

    d. Occasional rapid, jerky eye movement

2. When performing an otoscopic examination of a child who is crying, which of the following would the nurse identify as indicating a problem?

    a. Erythema of the tympanic membrane

    b. Gray appearance of the tympanic membrane

    c. Bubbles behind the tympanic membrane

    d. Movement of the tympanic membrane with pneumatic otoscopy

3. The nurse is listening to a 10-year-old child's heart sounds. At which of the following locations will the S1 heart sound be heard loudest?

    a. Aortic and pulmonary areas

    b. Tricuspid and mitral areas

    c. Erb's point

    d. Apical and aortic areas

4. When preparing to examine a toddler, which of the following would be most helpful in facilitating the examination?

    a. Let the child stay close to the parent

    b. Distract the child with a toy

    c. Ask the parent to leave the room

    d. Provide appropriate covering

5. The nurse is performing a behavioral assessment of a 10-month-old child during a physical examination. Which of the following would the nurse most likely expect to find?

   a. Positive tonic neck reflex

   b. Assistance needed to sit

   c. Walking with one hand held

   d. Waving bye-bye

6. The nurse is performing a physical examination for a 4-year-old girl and has become concerned that she is anemic. Which of the following assessment findings would support this concern?

   a. Cyanosis of the lips and mouth

   b. Concave finger nails

   c. Yellow tint to the skin

   d. Lack of skin turgor

7. The nurse is examining the internal nasal cavity of an uncooperative 3-year-old child. Which of the following would the nurse document as a normal finding?

   a. Grayish mucosa with clear discharge

   b. Bright red mucosa and purulent discharge

   c. Discharge from only one nostril

   d. Pink mucosa with watery discharge

8. When examining the mouth and throat of a 5-year-old child, which of the following would the nurse expect to find?

   a. Thin upper lip with long philtrum

   b. A tight frenulum

   c. Large tonsils with crypts

   d. Tonsillar exudate

Pharmacologic Management

Learning Objectives

- Discuss age-based variations in pharmacokinetics and pharmacodynamics.
- Describe safety measures to reduce the risk of error in administering medications to children.
- Explain developmentally appropriate techniques to administer medications via different routes to children.

SECTION I: ASSESSING YOUR UNDERSTANDING

Activity A *Fill in the blanks.*

1. _____ is the process that involves the absorption, distribution, metabolism, and elimination of drugs; it is the action of the body on the drug.

2. The measured or calculated surface of a human body, the area covered by skin is known as _____ _____ _____.

3. The actions of a drug or how a drug produces physiologic and biochemical changes at the cellular, tissue, and organ levels is known as _____.

4. The _____ route is the preferred route for medication administration in children.

5. The right _____ is the sixth medication right used with children.

6. _____ time is used for scheduling pediatric medications to help prevent medication errors.

7. A nurse should only take _____ medication orders during an emergency situation.

8. When administering a bad-tasting oral medication, offer the school-aged child an _____ _____ to suck on to help numb their mouth and consequently dull the taste.

Activity B *Match the developmental level of the child in column A with proper medication administration approach in column B.*

Column A	Column B
____ 1. Infancy	a. Give concrete explanations of the purpose of the medication.
____ 2. Early childhood	
____ 3. Middle childhood	b. Educate about safe self-medication.
____ 4. Adolescence	c. Place oral medication in a nipple.
	d. Explain in simple terms the reason for the medication.

Activity C *Write the correct sequence of medication administration in the boxes provided.*

1. The medication order is transcribed.
2. The drug is given to the patient.
3. The drug is dispensed.
4. The drug is calculated and prescribed.

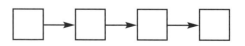

Activity D *Write the correct sequence of the administration of a topical medication.*

1. Cleanse the skin.

2. Assess the skin for an adverse drug reaction.

3. Assess the skin.

4. Apply the topical medication.

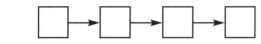

Activity E *Briefly answer the following.*

1. Name the six rights of medication administration and give a brief description of each.

   _____

   _____

   _____

2. List at least five key elements for medication administration in a nonmedical setting.

   _____

   _____

   _____

SECTION II: APPLYING YOUR KNOWLEDGE

Activity F *Consider the scenario and answer the questions.*

William is a 75-lb, 12-year-old boy admitted to the hospital for bronchiolitis and an asthma exacerbation. Today is day 2 of his hospital admission. The following is a list of his medication orders:

Zithromax: 500 mg orally on day 1, then 250 mg orally on days 2 through 5
Availability: Oral suspension, 200 mg/5 mL
Prednisone: 15 mg orally every 12 hours
Availability: Oral suspension, 5 mg/mL
Tylenol: 10 mg/kg orally every 4 to 6 hours PRN
Availability: Tablets, 80 mg, 160 mg, 325 mg, 650 mg

1. How many kilograms does William weigh?

   _____

2. How many milligrams of Zithromax will William receive today? _____

3. How many milliliters of Zithromax oral suspension would you give William today?

   _____

4. If your pediatric drug book states that the normal safe dose range for prednisone is 0.5 to 2 mg/kg/day in divided doses with a maximum of 20 to 40 mg/day, is this a safe dose for him? _____

5. William is asking for Tylenol because he is achy today. What is the dose in milligrams that you would give him? _____ How would you administer this dose in the tablets that are available? _____

SECTION III: PRACTICING FOR NCLEX

Activity G *Answer the following questions.*

1. Amanda is a new mom who has brought her 2-week-old infant in for his first checkup. Amanda is taking several daily medications and she is concerned about breast-feeding while taking them. Which of the following is the most appropriate response by the nurse?

   a. "Most medications are not excreted in breast milk, so it should not be a concern."

   b. "Are you telling me that you take medications every day and then breast-feed your infant?"

   c. "All medications are excreted differently in breast milk and affect your newborn differently. Let's take a look at *Medications and Mother's Milk* and then speak with the pediatrician."

   d. "We will send a sample of your breast milk to the lab to have it analyzed."

2. A nurse caring for a 5-year-old boy with asthma is preparing to administer an oral dose of a prescription drug. After checking that the name and dosage amount are correct, she looks up the normal dosage in a pediatric drug book. She determines that the dose ordered for her patient is much higher than the safe dose range in the book. What should she do next?

   a. Ask the patient's mother if this is a normal dose amount for him.

   b. Give the dose, since that is what is ordered.

   c. Call the practitioner who prescribed the medication to verify the dose.

   d. Call the nurse from the last shift and ask her if she gave the prescribed dose.

3. An every 6 hours PRN oral dose of Ibuprofen was given to a 6-month-old infant at 9 am. The infant spit up the medication along with some formula about 3 minutes later. What is the correct nursing response?

   a. Administer half the original dose, because since you don't know how much medication the infant absorbed.

   b. Give no more medication until the next dose is due to be given.

   c. Give a full dose of the medication in 3 hours instead of 6 hours when the next dose is due.

   d. Readminister the full dose because it was thrown up less than 5 minutes after administration.

4. At the end of the shift, a nurse discovers a medication error has been made. What is the correct action for the nurse to take first?

   a. Notify the prescriber and pharmacist immediately.

   b. Make a narrative note in the chart.

   c. Apologize to the patient.

   d. Correct the Medication Administration Record.

5. When administering a medication to a child, which of the following approaches is more suitable?

   a. Pretend the medicine is a "yummy" treat.

   b. Ask the parents what has worked best in the past.

   c. "Reward" the child's good behavior with their medication.

   d. Administer the medication as quickly as possible to minimize resistance.

6. When administering oral medication to an infant, what is the best method of administration?

   a. Place the medication in a small measuring cup and slowly pour it into the infant's mouth.

   b. Squirt a small amount in the side of the infant's cheek and allow the infant to swallow before squirting more.

   c. Mix the medication in the infant's formula or cereal.

   d. Hold the infant's nose and squirt the medicine down the back on the tongue.

7. When administering an intramuscular (IM) injection to a 1-year-old child, which of the following is the best method of administration?

   a. Discourage the child from crying or acting out.

   b. Use the vastus lateralis as an acceptable site.

   c. Use the dorsogluteal muscle as an acceptable site.

   d. Use a 25G needle.

8. When administering a rectal medication to a 3-year-old child, which of the following is the most appropriate nursing intervention?

   a. Place the child on his back and bring both knees to the chest.

   b. Use petrolatum jelly to lubricate the medication.

   c. Have the child pant like a puppy to help relax the anal sphincter and distract them.

   d. If needed, cut the suppository crosswise to increase absorption.

9. Austin is a 2-year-old child due to have ear drops administered by the nurse. Which of the following demonstrates the proper technique to administer this medication?

   a. Place the child in a supine position and turn his head to one side, then pull the ear up and back to administer the medication.

   b. Remove the medication from the refrigerator and immediately administer the medication.

   c. Place the child in a supine position and turn his head to one side, then pull the ear down and back to administer the medication.

   d. Tilt the head to expose the ear upward, then place the dropper against the outer ear canal to stabilize it while administering the medication.

10. When administering ophthalmic medication to a 10-year-old child, which of the following demonstrates proper technique by the nurse?

    a. Position the child on his back and place a drop of medication directly onto the cornea.

    b. Position the child on his back and place your dominant hand on his forehead, then pull back the lower eyelid and place a drop of medication on the conjunctival sac.

    c. Have the child remain on his back with his eyes closed for 5 minutes after medication has been given.

    d. Gently cleanse the eye with a cotton ball soaked in normal saline and work from the outer to the inner canthus.

11. The nurse is preparing to administer one Prevacid tablet, 15 mg orally, to her 6-year-old female patient. Which of the following is the best nursing approach to use with this patient?

    a. Ask the patient whether she would like juice or water to take the medicine.

    b. Ask the patient if she is ready for her medication now.

    c. Use abstract rationales when explaining the use of the medication.

    d. Explain to her that taking medications is just like eating candy.

12. The nurse is preparing to give a 6-month-old infant an oral dose of amoxicillin. Which of the following is the best approach for the nurse to take when giving this medication?

    a. Position the child supine in the bed and stabilize the child's head with the nondominant hand as you give the medication.

    b. Explain to the child the need for the medication in simple terms.

    c. Ask the parents to leave the room when you administer this medication.

    d. Use an oral syringe and squirt a small amount of medicine at a time beside the tongue as you hold the child in your lap. Laying a child on their back to take oral medication can put them at risk for aspiration.

13. Alex is a 28-lb 2-year-old child with a medication order for ibuprofen, 5 mg/kg/dose. The ibuprofen that is stocked on the unit is a suspension of 100 mg/5 mL. How many milliliters would you give this patient?

    a. 140

    b. 64

    c. 3.18

    d. 31.8

14. You are caring for a 14-year-old patient in the hospital. During your assessment, the patient's pediatrician comes in for a visit. The patient asks her doctor if she can have something stronger for the pain she is experiencing. The doctor asks the nurse to write an order for morphine 4 mg IV every 4 to 6 hours for pain. Which of the following is the correct response for the nurse to give?

    a. "Yes, I will write a verbal order for morphine, 4 mg IV, every 4 to 6 hours for pain."

    b. "You will need to write the order in the chart. It is hospital policy to write verbal orders only in an emergency."

    c. "I can't do that."

    d. "Are you certain you want to give the patient something that strong?"

15. The nurse enters the room to administer an oral medication to an 18-month-old child. The mother is present in the room and asks the nurse which medication she is giving. The nurse responds with "amoxicillin; her antibiotic." The mom states that the child has thrown up the entire dose of this medication the past two times it was given. Which of the following is the best response for the nurse to give to the mother?

    a. "I will call the doctor and let him know your concerns before we give this dose."

    b. "I will ask the doctor about changing the medication during rounds later today. Let's give this dose because it is due now."

    c. "Let's see what happens after I give this dose."

    d. "Why don't you try to give this next dose?"

10

Pain Management

Learning Objectives

- Explain the physiologic mechanisms that lead to the sensation of pain.
- Identify factors that may intensify or modulate the pain experience.
- Discuss the assessment techniques and tools used to evaluate pain in children.
- Describe pharmacologic interventions used to manage pain in children.
- Describe biobehavioral nursing interventions to control pain and anxiety in children.
- Contrast manifestations of chronic pain with acute pain and how management strategies for children in special pain situations may differ.
- Discuss the role of the nurse on the interdisciplinary pain team.

SECTION I: ASSESSING YOUR UNDERSTANDING

Activity A *Fill in the blanks.*

1. The activity produced in the nervous system by noxious, potentially tissue-damaging, stimuli is known as _____.

2. The impaired sensitivity to touch, such as paresthesia and cutaneous hypesthesia is _____.

3. _____ is excessive sensation from pain.

4. When nonpainful stimuli, such as light touch, is perceived as painful, it is called _____.

5. _____ is one of the most widely accepted indicators of pain in infants.

6. _____ therapy involves combining analgesics so that less of each individual medication is required to relieve pain, and the potential for side effects therefore is less than it would be with single-agent therapy.

7. The _____ route is the preferred analgesia route used for children.

8. Children who report decreasing pain relief from previously effective doses of opioids may be experiencing _____ to the analgesic effects of the opioid and may therefore require a different dosage or another drug.

9. _____ of lidocaine uses an electrical field to drive local anesthetics across intact skin.

10. Pain that persists a month beyond the usual expected disease or injury course is considered to be _____.

11. Assessment of pain by nurses is performed most consistently when pain is viewed as the _____ _____ _____.

Activity B *Match the types of analgesia medication administration in column A with their disadvantages in column B.*

Column A	Column B
____ 1. Oral/PO	a. Oversedation
____ 2. Intravenous (IV)	b. Few available, very slow onset of action

_____ **3.** Intramuscular (IM)

_____ **4.** Subcutaneous (SQ)

_____ **5.** Transdermal

_____ **6.** Transmucosal

_____ **7.** Rectal

_____ **8.** Authorized agent-controlled analgesia (AACA)

_____ **9.** Patient-controlled analgesia (PCA)

_____ **10.** Intraspinal

for opioids (12–16 hours)

c. Hypotension, bradycardia, apnea, and motor blockade may occur

d. Fluctuations in absorption rates, delayed peak (30–60 minutes), and rapid falloff

e. Not well accepted by children; absorption varies

f. PCA by proxy, oversedation, constant titration

g. Slow absorption, less acceptable to children because it involves the use of a needle

h. Increased incidence of adverse side effects

i. Noxious taste and burning sensation

j. Delayed onset of action (45 minutes), delayed peak effect (1–2 hours), and noxious taste

Activity C _Write the correct sequence of nociception in the boxes provided._

1. Transduction

2. Perception

3. Modulation

4. Transmission

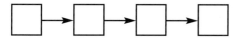

Activity D _Briefly answer the following._

1. List the three types of pain relief medications given to children, and describe their indications for use and their differences.

     a. _____

     b. _____

     c. _____

_____

_____

_____

2. List the four stages of nociception and give a brief description of each stage.

     a. _____

     b. _____

     c. _____

     d. _____

_____

_____

_____

SECTION II: APPLYING YOUR KNOWLEDGE

Activity E _Consider the scenario and answer the questions._

Aiden is a 9-year-old postoperative appendectomy patient who is being discharged from the hospital. His parents are in the room awaiting discharge teaching.

1. How would you teach the parents to determine the pain level of their child?

_____

_____

2. What information would you be certain to include when teaching the parents about pain medication administration?

_____

_____

SECTION III: PRACTICING FOR NCLEX

Activity F *Answer the following questions.*

1. Developmentally appropriate pain intensity scales can be used to obtain a self-report from children as young as _____ year(s) of age.
   a. 1
   b. 2
   c. 3
   d. 4

2. By _____ years of age, children have learned to control their facial expressions and may mask facial indications of pain.
   a. 4
   b. 5
   c. 6
   d. 3

3. Which of the following lists the best physical indicators of stress in a preterm newborn?
   a. Crying, arm and leg flexion, and facial grimace
   b. Gaze aversion, hiccups, yawning, and flaccid posture
   c. Lying still, rigid, or curled in a fetal position; guarding or touching the painful area; and clenching fists
   d. Crying, moaning, refusal to move, decreased appetite, irritability, and sleep disturbance

4. Derek is a 4-year-old cancer patient. The nurse is preparing Derek's parents for a painful procedure. Which of the following is the best statement for the nurse to make?
   a. "Derek won't need any pain medication because the procedure is a quick one."
   b. "You will need to leave the room during the procedure."
   c. "Your presence during the procedure will only make matters worse for Derek."
   d. "Derek will receive pain medication before the procedure and you may stay with him during the procedure. Here are a few suggestions to help him through the procedure."

5. James is a 16-year-old sickle cell patient just admitted to the hospital for treatment of a sickle cell crisis. It is time for insertion of an IV. What is the best distraction technique for the nurse to utilize during this procedure?
   a. Ask James to count to 100 out loud.
   b. Have an aide read him a story during the procedure.
   c. Provide James with a video game to play during the procedure.
   d. Provide James with a bubble machine during the procedure.

6. Patti is a 10-year-old patient being seen at a clinic for a wellness checkup. After hearing she is due for an immunization (injection) today, Patti is visibly agitated and upset. Which of the following is the best relaxation technique the nurse can use to prepare Patti for the injection?
   a. Have Patti breathe in deeply through her nose and breathe out slowly through her mouth five times before the injection.
   b. Play loud music with an upbeat tempo.
   c. Turn off all the lights so Patti is unable to see the injection.
   d. Tell Patti to relax and pretend she is at the beach.

7. Which of the following positioning techniques is most appropriate for a newborn receiving an IV in the scalp?
   a. Place the newborn in a supine position and restrain the hands and feet away from the body.
   b. Allow for freedom of movement of the newborn's extremities during the procedure.
   c. Bundle the infant in a blanket to reduce the amount of extremity movement, and provide facilitative tucking during the procedure.
   d. Have another care provider hold the infant's arms and legs against the bed during the procedure.

8. Which of the following is the best method of reducing pain during an IM injection to a child?

    a. Application of a heat pack for 20 minutes prior to the injection.

    b. Gentle massage of the muscle for 10 minutes prior to the injection.

    c. Application of an ice pack for 30 minutes prior to the injection.

    d. Ice cube massage for a few minutes just prior to the injection.

9. Which of the following nursing interventions should be completed when caring for a child who is sedated?

    a. Monitor vital signs every 2 minutes and evaluate oxygen saturation every 10 minutes.

    b. Monitor vital signs and level of consciousness every 5 minutes and place the child on a continuous cardiac and oxygen saturation monitor.

    c. Monitor vital signs and level of consciousness every 15 minutes.

    d. Monitor vital signs and level of consciousness every 20 to 30 minutes and place child on a continuous cardiac monitor.

10. Stephanie is a 12-year-old child being seen in the emergency department after a motor vehicle accident. After the ABCs have been addressed, the nurse moves on to assess "D," or discomfort. Which of the following is the best nursing intervention to implement after discovering Stephanie is in severe pain?

    a. Administer opioid pain medication immediately.

    b. Assess the patient for shock or head injury before administering opioid medications.

    c. Administer only nonopioid medications in the emergency department.

    d. Obtain parental permission before administering any opioid medications in the emergency department.

11. Which of the following medications is most useful for children with rheumatoid arthritis?

    a. Aspirin

    b. Ibuprofen

    c. Tylenol

    d. Tylenol with codeine

12. Which of the following pain assessment tools is most appropriate for a 5-year-old postoperative patient?

    a. Pain diary

    b. Numeric rating scale

    c. Faces pain scale

    d. Visual analogue scale

13. Which of the following pain assessment tools is most appropriate for a 10-year-old patient with cerebral palsy who is severely developmentally delayed and nonverbal?

    a. Faces pain scale

    b. Numeric rating scale.

    c. FLACC pain rating scale.

    d. Varni-Thompson Pediatric Pain Questionnaire

14. When caring for a 14-year-old patient in chronic pain, which analgesic medication would be most beneficial to the patient when attempting to control pain at the modulation stage?

    a. Ibuprofen

    b. Morphine sulfate

    c. Baclofen

    d. Tylenol with codeine

Activity G *Choose all answers that apply.*

1. Which of the following assessment findings are common with children who experience chronic pain? (Choose all that apply.)

    a. Normal vital signs

    b. Developmental regression

    c. Depression

    d. Disrupted sleep patterns

2. When considering the developmental level of a preschooler, which of the following behaviors would the nurse most likely observe? (Choose all that apply.)

    a. Fears bodily injury or mutilation

    b. Lacks words for pain

    c. Needs some control over the situation

    d. Can delay gratification

3. Which of the following is true of preterm infants and how they experience pain? (Choose all that apply.)

    a. Their facial features include a grimace, clenched teeth, tightly shut lips or biting lips, wide open eyes, and a wrinkled forehead.

    b. Their cry has more characteristics that arouse a listener, it is higher pitched, and it is often of shorter duration.

    c. They have less vigorous movements and they are often limp, flaccid, or listless.

    d. They exhibit withdrawal of a limb and posture that is rigid posture, guarded, or flaccid.

4. Which of the following would indicate a child is suitable to receive patient-controlled analgesia (PCA)? (Choose all that apply.)

    a. The child is able to quantify pain.

    b. The child is unable to tolerate oral analgesics.

    c. The child understands the relation between pushing the button and receiving medication.

    d. The child reports unsatisfactory pain relief with the current regimen.

5. Which of the following are common opioid side effects that should be monitored by the nurse? (Choose all that apply.)

    a. Pruritus

    b. Nausea and vomiting

    c. Diarrhea

    d. Urinary retention

C H A P T E R

11

Acute Illness as a Challenge to Health Maintenance

Learning Objectives

- Facilitate care during acute illness to minimize stress for the child and family.
- Discuss the impact of hospitalization on the child's and family's coping and adaptation responses.
- Select nursing interventions to provide basic care needs for the child during an episode of acute illness.
- Select interventions that provide psychosocial support to the family during hospitalization.
- Describe nursing care of the child having surgery.
- Identify factors that prepare the child and family for a smooth transition from the acute care environment to a community setting.

SECTION I: ASSESSING YOUR UNDERSTANDING

Activity A *Fill in the blanks.*

1. An _____ _____ is a threat to a child and his or her family characterized by suddenness, severity, and disruption of the normal patterns of everyday life.

2. _____ care is provision of care in a manner that that minimizes the emotional and physical threat to the child.

3. The actions used to restrict activity as part of the treatment plan (e.g., traction); to prevent interfering with tubes, dressings, or healing tissue (e.g., elbow immobilizers); or to facilitate administration of medications or treatments is called _____.

4. The most important way to minimize exposure to and transmission of pathogens is by following _____ _____.

5. Do not perform any uncomfortable or painful procedures (such as an injection) in the _____ to promote the child's perception that, within the confines of this room, they are safe from intrusion and discomfort as much as possible.

6. _____ _____ _____ is the purposeful use of animals to provide affection, attention, diversion, and relaxation.

7. _____ _____ are used to prevent the child from reaching the face to do harm by preventing elbow flexion while leaving the hands free for play and exploration.

8. _____ _____ is useful when performing procedures for which the infant or toddler must remain still.

9. A _____ _____ is a legal document that gives doctors and other hospital personnel permission to care for a child in the hospital.

10. Children with asthma are at risk for _____ during surgery.

41

Activity B *Match the types of atraumatic care nursing interventions in column A with the aspect of care they focus on in column B.*

Column A

_____ 1. Medicate freely

_____ 2. Prepare a child prior to with a visit

_____ 3. Use topical anesthesia prior to by injecting the area with an intradermal anesthetic

_____ 4. Keep as non-threatening as possible

_____ 5. Use a topical anesthetic and attempt to place in a location where the child or infant will not need a lot of restraints or arm boards

_____ 6. Use a topical anesthetic prior to and use the appropriate length and bore needle

_____ 7. Always explain what is happening to the child—in his or her terms, not in adult and medical terms

_____ 8. Use as minimally as possible and use the least restrictive one that provides safety

_____ 9. Apply a topical anesthetic and perform as infrequently as possible

Column B

a. Psychological

b. Environment

c. Restraints

d. Pain

e. Surgery

f. Suturing

g. Blood draws

h. IVs

i. Injections

Activity C *Write the correct sequence of patient education in the boxes provided.*

1. Evaluation of the effectiveness of the teaching plan

2. Assessment of the problem and of readiness to learn

3. Development of a teaching plan

4. Implementation of the teaching plan

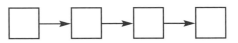

Activity D *Briefly answer the following.*

1. List and describe the three phases a child goes through when experiencing separation from a parent.

_____

_____

_____

2. What nursing interventions would be best when a parent is unable to visit a child in the hospital?

_____

_____

_____

3. Name three advantages of a care conference.

_____

_____

_____

SECTION II: APPLYING YOUR KNOWLEDGE

Activity E *Consider the scenario and answer the questions.*

Andrea is a 3-year-old child who had just been admitted to the preoperative area for an abdominal hernia repair. Her parents are with her and both look very anxious.

1. What are some nursing interventions you could implement to help alleviate the parents' anxiety?

_____

_____

2. Andrea needs an IV inserted before surgery. What developmental considerations would you use when explaining the procedure to her and when performing the procedure?

_____

_____

3. What postoperative instructions would you give to the parents before discharging the child?

_____

_____

SECTION III: PRACTICING FOR NCLEX

Activity F *Choose all answers that apply.*

1. Which of the following nursing interventions best demonstrates family-centered care?
   a. Extended visitation hours from 6:00 AM until 11:00 PM
   b. Liberal, 24-hour-a-day visitation policy
   c. Weekly patient care conferences
   d. An expectation that the family will provide the patient's care around the clock

2. When preparing to bathe a 6-month-old infant in the hospital with an IV, which of the following is the most effective nursing intervention?
   a. Determine whether the infant can stand unassisted.
   b. Bathe the infant daily at the same time of the day.
   c. Ask the parent whether the infant is routinely bathed in the morning or the evening.
   d. Discourage parents from bathing the infant to prevent the IV from being dislodged.

3. When providing oral hygiene to a 4-year-old hospitalized patient, which of the following is the best approach to take?
   a. Allow the 4-year-old to brush his teeth unassisted.
   b. Provide a fluoride rinse after brushing.
   c. Allow the 4-year-old to use a toothbrush from home.
   d. Use a soft cloth or sponge to clean the gums.

4. The nurse enters a hospital room and finds her 14-year-old patient dressed in clothing from home. Which of the following statements is most appropriate for the nurse to make to the patient?
   a. "You should really wear the hospital gowns during your stay; they are much cleaner than the clothes you brought from home."
   b. "You are welcome to wear whatever is the most comfortable for you while you are in the hospital."
   c. "I wouldn't wear your own clothing while you are here; they may become stained."
   d. "Please put the hospital gown on."

5. Which of the following nursing interventions will help decrease anxiety and embarrassment when assisting an adolescent with toileting while in the hospital?
   a. Encourage them to express feelings of embarrassment and anxiety.
   b. Store urinals and bedpans close to the bedside.
   c. Allow adolescents to complete all toileting needs without assistance.
   d. Allow for as much privacy as possible and be direct and matter-of-fact.

6. When caring for a 3-month-old infant, which of the following shows the correct position to place the child for sleep?
   a. Supine with no soft bedding or toys in the crib
   b. Supine with blankets placed under and on top of the infant
   c. Prone with no soft bedding or toys in the crib
   d. Prone with the head of the bed elevated

7. When caring for a child in the hospital, which of the following is the best nursing intervention to prevent sleep disturbance?
   a. Obtain vital signs based on hospital routine and put the child to bed after completed.
   b. Keep lights low during the day and at night.
   c. Assess the sleep and nap routines used at home, and organize care around those sleep times.
   d. Inform parents of procedure times and have them organize the child's sleep around them.

8. Which of the following demonstrates proper identification in the acute care setting?

   a. "Hello. Is your name Angie?"

   b. Verify the child's identity using a birth date and complete name, and match it to a medication order.

   c. Verify the child's identity using a birth date and a room number, and match it to a laboratory requisition slip.

   d. Verify the child's identity by asking a parent who the child is and matching it to a medication administration record.

9. Which of the following demonstrates proper use of restraints in the acute care setting?

   a. Placing a child in a restraint as a form of punishment for unacceptable behavior

   b. Placing the child in the least restrictive method of restraint as possible

   c. Securing a limb immobilizer to the side rail of the bed

   d. Use of restraints is unacceptable in any acute care setting

10. Which one of the following demonstrates the proper technique for transporting patients in the acute care setting?

    a. Have the patient walk to the radiology department located on the opposite end of the hospital.

    b. Bundle the newborn patient in a blanket and carry the patient to the laboratory.

    c. Use a wheelchair to transport a teenage patient to the surgery department.

    d. Leave the patient in the waiting room as you walk back to the treatment area to check them in.

11. Which of the following is the best nursing intervention when preventing latex allergies?

    a. Identify those at risk for latex allergies.

    b. Use nonlatex gloves.

    c. Use nonlatex IV tubing.

    d. Draw up medications into syringes just prior to giving them.

12. Which of the following is true of child abductions? (Choose all that apply.)

    a. Most of the missing children in the United States are abducted by one of their parents.

    b. A well-planned and structured infant and child security program can prevent child abductions in the acute care setting.

    c. Visitor identification is a key way to keep children safe from abduction in the acute care setting.

    d. Abductions can occur in the acute care setting.

13. Which of the following statements is an accurate description of separation anxiety?

    a. Separation anxiety resolves as soon as the parent returns.

    b. Separation anxiety occurs only in children 6 months to 4 years old.

    c. The adolescent suffers separation anxiety when separated from peers rather than parents.

    d. Separation anxiety can be described as having four phases or stages.

14. Which of the following are considered to be acceptable coping strategies to be utilized in the acute care setting? (Choose all that apply.)

    a. Play

    b. Drawing pictures

    c. Music

    d. Tearing up old bandages

15. Which of the following statements about sibling visitation in the hospital is accurate?

    a. Hospital visits should be discouraged for siblings to reduce exposure to diseases.

    b. Sibling visitation is beneficial for the entire family and can help maintain a sense of normalcy and routine while in the hospital.

    c. Sibling visitation can lead to feelings of jealousy.

    d. Sibling visitation can lead to confusion and misunderstandings about the hospitalized child.

16. Which of the following are accurate statements concerning surgery and children? (Choose all that apply.)

    a. Children's preoperative anxiety is related to their parents' preoperative anxiety.

    b. Preoperative anxiety exists only in the adult setting.

    c. Preoperative anxiety can be reduced with presurgery education.

    d. Tours and videos are helpful to educate children about surgery and what to expect while in the hospital.

17. When obtaining an informed consent, which of the following is true?

    a. Emergency procedures must have a signed consent before they are performed on a child.

    b. A biologic parent is the only person authorized to sign a consent form for a child.

    c. A parent or legal guardian may sign a consent form for a child.

    d. A patient can be admitted to the hospital without a signed consent form.

18. Children with neuromuscular disorders may be at risk for which of the following during surgery?

    a. Postoperative apnea during the first 6 months of life

    b. Increased intracranial pressure as a result of cerebral vasodilation during induction

    c. Bronchospasm

    d. Anesthesia-related cardiac arrest

19. Prolonged hospitalization can have negative effects on a child. Which of the following nursing interventions can help minimize these negative effects? (Choose all that apply.)

    a. Early developmental intervention

    b. Consistent caregivers

    c. Taking infants to the playroom

    d. Providing school for older children

20. Which of the following nursing interventions would be the most beneficial for the child who is being discharged after a long hospitalization?

    a. Make a follow-up appointment.

    b. Have the parents sign the discharge forms.

    c. Have the parents complete a satisfaction survey.

    d. Have the parents assume total care of the child in the hospital for 24 hours.

12

Chronic Conditions as a Challenge to Health Maintenance

Learning Objectives

- Define *chronic condition*.
- Discuss the broad spectrum of disorders that can be defined as chronic conditions.
- Discuss reasons for the disparity in determining the prevalence of children with chronic conditions. Analyze the impact of chronic conditions on children and families.
- Understand interventions to promote health and normalization for children with chronic conditions and their families.
- Discuss issues related to having a child with a chronic condition.
- Contrast pediatric rehabilitation and habilitation from adult rehabilitation.
- Delineate nursing interventions and strategies to assist the child in gaining independence during the rehabilitative and habilitative processes.
- Discuss the impact of having a chronic condition on the child/adolescent.
- Discuss the advocacy role of the nurse related to the laws protecting children and adolescents with chronic conditions.
- Describe nursing strategies to improve the transition from pediatric settings to adult services.

SECTION I: ASSESSING YOUR UNDERSTANDING

Activity A *Match the terms in column A with the description or related statement from column B.*

Column A

_____ 1. Mainstream

_____ 2. Remission

_____ 3. Chronic illness

_____ 4. Handicap

_____ 5. The child with diabetes

Column B

a. Integration into the regular classroom setting

b. Limitation imposed by society

c. Person-first language

d. No symptoms evident

e. Implication of being sick and needing to recover

Activity B *Fill in the blanks.*

1. Cystic fibrosis affects _____ organ systems.

2. Ulcerative colitis alternates between periods of remission and _____.

3. Some chronic conditions are secondary to or occur as a _____ of another risk factor.

4. It is often not until _____ that young children born with chronic conditions begin to perceive difference between themselves and their peers.

5. Adolescents with chronic conditions are often treated like _____ children.

Activity C *Supply the information requested.*

1. The following terms are related to chronicity. Label each as either an appropriate term or one to be avoided.

   a. Chronic illness _____

   b. The diabetic _____

   c. The child with cystic fibrosis _____

   d. Children with special healthcare needs _____

   e. Handicap _____

   f. Impaired children _____

   g. Chronic condition _____

   h. Retarded _____

   i. Slow _____

2. Disability has at least two official definitions. Describe the ADA definition of disability and the IDEA definition of disability.

3. Explain the difference between chronic illness and chronic condition.

SECTION II: APPLYING YOUR KNOWLEDGE

Activity D *Consider the scenario and answer the questions.*

Mary Andrews brings her 14-year-old daughter Melissa to the clinic for a checkup. Melissa was diagnosed with Crohn's disease 1 year ago. During the past year, she has become more symptomatic and has required a more complicated medication regime and dietary restrictions, and has missed a total of 2 weeks from school. The realization that Melissa has a chronic condition and its effect on her daily living and her family is becoming more apparent. Melissa's mother verbalizes concern over Melissa's absenteeism and the cost of the medication. Melissa loves to play tennis and is

concerned that she will not be able to play on the tennis team in the fall.

1. What implications does Melissa's chronic condition have for the nurse caring for her?

   _____

   _____

2. How would the nurse advocate for Melissa?

   _____

   _____

SECTION III: PRACTICING FOR NCLEX

Activity E *Choose the answer that is the best answer for each question.*

1. The parents of a 12-year-old boy with Duchenne muscular dystrophy are talking to the nurse who assists their son's healthcare provider. They are expressing feelings of powerlessness because of their lack of ability to control the progression of their son's condition. They feel that the progression is somehow their fault. Which of the following should the nurse say?

   a. "Your feelings are normal; it is OK to talk about this."

   b. "You are doing a great job with his care."

   c. "What do you think you are you doing wrong?"

   d. "Why don't you talk to the doctor about this?"

2. A nurse who is caring for a 10-year-old boy with a recent tracheostomy is teaching the parents how to use the respiratory suction pump in preparation for the child's discharge from the hospital. Which question would be most important for the nurse to ask the parents first?

   a. "Do you think you will be able to do this?"

   b. "Do you know what this suction pump device is?"

   c. "Do you understand why your son needs this respiratory suction pump?"

   d. "Do you have any concerns about this respiratory suction pump?"

3. The nurse has been caring for an 11-year-old boy who requires extensive home care. The parents have indicated that they are feeling tired, both physically and emotionally. Which of the following actions would the nurse do first to provide relief for the parents?

   a. Refer the parents to respite care providers

   b. Encourage the parents to discuss their feelings

   c. Identify past coping mechanisms

   d. Determine the family's expectations of siblings

4. The nurse is assessing the progress of a 12-year-old girl with a permanent tracheostomy and her family in coping with her disability. Which of the following indicates the child and family are demonstrating successful coping?

   a. The girl wears in-style, fashionable clothing

   b. The girl's respirator is on her bedside table

   c. The parents limit socializing outside of the home

   d. The parents are permissive with the girl

5. The nurse is caring for an 11-year-old girl with diabetes. She is teaching the girl and her parents how to operate her new insulin pump. Which of the following is the best way to present new material to the child and her parents?

   a. Hands-on demonstrations and practice sessions

   b. Developmentally appropriate reading material

   c. Video presentations with practice sessions

   d. Multiple developmentally appropriate methods

6. The nurse knows that children with chronic conditions have a wide variety of needs that must be met. Which of the following is most easily overlooked?

   a. Providing adequate transportation for equipment

   b. Acknowledging developmental accomplishments

   c. Managing discomfort during routine procedures

   d. Scheduling a physical examination once a year

CHAPTER 13

Palliative Care

Learning Objectives

- Relate the sociopolitical influences on the development of palliative care services for children.
- State the core definitions and principles of palliative care.
- Describe models used to guide palliative care services.
- Delineate barriers to implementation of pediatric palliative care.
- Select strategies that enhance communication during the provision of palliative care.
- Identify interdisciplinary measures to promote quality of life at end of life.
- Describe interdisciplinary care interventions at the time death occurs.
- Examine the process of grief and bereavement in the family coping with the death of a child.
- Describe bereavement responses of children when a loved one dies.
- Explain support measures that healthcare providers can implement as they grieve the loss of a pediatric patient.

SECTION I: ASSESSING YOUR UNDERSTANDING

Activity A Fill in the blanks.

1. Approximately _____ of children in the United States have a chronic or debilitating illness.

2. The actions to relieve symptoms or an approach that improves quality of life in patients and families facing life-threatening illnesses is known as _____
_____.

3. _____ is a form of healthcare that provides palliative care services across a variety of settings, based on the philosophy that death is a natural part of the life cycle.

4. _____ is never used for long-term pain control because of the resultant accumulation of a toxic metabolite after as few as 3 days of treatment.

5. The child must be in the terminal phase of illness, usually with death expected during the ensuing _____, to qualify for hospice care.

6. _____ _____ allows the parents and family to leave the child with the assistance of a home health aide or hospice volunteer.

7. _____ is the painful, sad, and anguished feeling accompanying loss.

8. The mental work following any loss, which allows adaptation to that loss is called _____.

9. Be certain to involve the _____ of the child that is dying in the daily care and activities surrounding that child.

10. Advanced directives of a child younger than 18 years of age are not followed if a _____ does not agree with them.

Activity B Match the types of grief in column A with their definition in column B.

Column A	Column B
____ 1. Anticipatory	a. Uncomplicated grief reactions that are suppressed or postponed
____ 2. Uncomplicated	
____ 3. Chronic	

49

____ **4.** Delayed

____ **5.** Exaggerated

____ **6.** Masked

b. The survivor is not aware that behaviors that interfere with normal functioning are a result of the loss

c. Also known as "normal" grief

d. Anticipated and real losses associated with diagnosis, acute and chronic illnesses, and terminal illness

e. Grief reactions that do not subside and continue over very long periods of time

f. Survivor resorts to self-destructive behaviors such as suicide

Activity C *Write the correct sequence of the five stages of grief according to Kubler-Ross.*

1. Depression

2. Bargaining

3. Denial

4. Acceptance

5. Anger

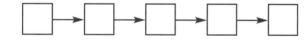

Activity D *Briefly answer the following.*

1. List at least four conditions in which the need for palliative care exists among children.

_____

_____

_____

2. List the five core principals from which palliative care must be integrated throughout the trajectory of a child's illness according to Last Acts.

_____

_____

_____

3. Name the four cornerstones of clinical practice in pediatric palliative care identified by the Initiative for Pediatric Palliative Care (IPPC).

_____

_____

_____

SECTION II: APPLYING YOUR KNOWLEDGE

Activity E *Consider the scenario and answer the questions.*

Tim and Jennifer Schneider have just learned that their 10-year-old son, John, is losing his fight with cancer and has approximately 2 months left to live. He has a 4-year-old younger brother named Jack and a 12-year-old sister name Samantha. The family is all present in a conference room at a local children's hospital. John immediately expresses his wish to return home.

1. After a long discussion with John, the parents ask if he can be released and taken home. What do you tell them?

_____

_____

2. What resource would benefit the Schneider family the best at this point?

_____

_____

3. After John and the siblings have left the room, Jennifer and Tim ask what they should do with Samantha and Jack. What would you tell them?

_____

_____

SECTION III: PRACTICING FOR NCLEX

Activity F *Choose all answers that apply.*

1. Which of the following best describes the Initiative for Pediatric Palliative Care's (IPPC) third cornerstone?
   a. The extreme vulnerability of the dying child and the family imposes an ethical claim on the healthcare providers.
   b. It expresses the need to reflect on one's own culture as well as the culture of the child and the family.
   c. This concept reflects the importance of constant evaluation of one's beliefs and how those beliefs are translated into palliative care practices.
   d. Clinical practice in pediatric palliative care is fundamentally relational, involving a "two-way" relationship with the child and the family.

2. When dealing with a grieving family, which of the following statements is accurate?
   a. The nurse must keep an "emotional distance" from the family during the process of grieving.
   b. The nurse should focus on the individual family members.
   c. Focus should be centered on adding years to the child's life.
   d. Establish a relationship, by being present both physically and emotionally, and by continuing to focus on the family as a system.

3. Which of the following statements best describes the barriers to implementing palliative care?
   a. The child's wished are carried out despite the barriers involved.
   b. There is often disparity between the way children die and the way they want to be cared for when dying.
   c. Most families accept the reality of the dying child with little difficulty.
   d. Healthcare providers are well-educated on the process of death and dying.

4. What percentage of children receive hospice care that could benefit from it?
   a. 25%
   b. 10%
   c. 5%
   d. 1%

5. At what developmental age does a child understand that death is permanent and irreversible?
   a. Preschool
   b. Early adolescence
   c. School age
   d. Late adolescence

6. When caring for a terminal child, which of the following statements concerning anorexia is accurate?
   a. Be vigilant in offering the dying child food and fluids.
   b. Absence of food and fluids in the dying child can cause additional pain.
   c. Enteral or parenteral feedings should be initiated when the dying child suffers from anorexia.
   d. Anorexia experienced in the dying child does not cause additional suffering.

7. Haley is a 13-year-old child who is terminally ill with cancer. She expresses a desire to continue school to her mother while you are present. Her mom looks to you for advice. What is the best nursing response?
   a. "School will be physically and mentally exhausting for you at this time. It would not be a good idea for you."
   b. "That is completely your parents' decision to make."
   c. "I think that is a good idea. We should discuss that with your parents and your doctor to make arrangements."
   d. "Why would you want to spend what little time you have left in school?"

8. When caring for a terminally ill child in the last stages of the death process, which of the following is an omission that might be made?
   a. Antibiotics to treat a urinary tract infection
   b. Discontinuing parenteral or enteral nutrition even if the child is hungry
   c. Daily weights and lab work
   d. Suctioning and oxygen therapy

9. When preparing for the parents' final visit with the child who has died unexpectedly, which of the following is the best nursing intervention?

a. Prepare the parents for what the child will look like, especially if extensive injuries are involved.

b. Tidy the room by removing all traces of resuscitative equipment.

c. Dim the lights in order that the harsh reality of the child's death might be softened.

d. Do not encourage a parent to visit the dead child if they do not wish to do so.

10. Which of the following statements best describes the correct sibling involvement in a child's death?

a. The sibling should attend the child's funeral, even if they do not wish to do so.

b. The child should have an adult appointed to attend to them during the funeral.

c. The sibling should not be included in the preparation of the service because of the emotional trauma they might endure.

d. Siblings should be protected from the death process.

11. Nancy has just experienced the loss of her 22-week preterm infant. Which of the following is the best nursing intervention for Nancy at this time?

a. Ask Nancy's husband if it is okay for her to see and hold the child.

b. Remind Nancy that she has three healthy children at home.

c. Bathe, then dress the infant and wrap him in a blanket before bringing him to the mother to hold.

d. If the parents do not wish to see the infant, encourage them to do so.

12. Which of the following are considered to be bereavement tasks? (Choose all that apply.)

a. Reacting to the separation

b. Recollecting and reexperiencing the deceased and the relationship

c. Reinvesting in the new world

d. Recognizing the loss

13. Which of the following are helpful suggestions to give to family and friends of the family that has experienced the death of a child? (Choose all that apply.)

a. Protect or shield the family from the reality of the situation.

b. Give a hug or a hand to hold.

c. Talk about the child.

d. Say you are sorry.

14. John is a 6-year-old terminally ill child who is in the last stages of dying. What nursing interventions are helpful when he begins agonal breaths? (Choose all that apply.)

a. Elevate the head of the bed.

b. Reassure the family present.

c. Provide a quiet and calm environment.

d. Gentle massage.

15. Which of the following are appropriate nursing interventions for a sibling of a deceased child? (Choose all that apply.)

a. Let the sibling know that feeling sad, angry, or scared is okay for adults and for children, and that crying is okay (even for boys).

b. Involve siblings in family discussions about the dying child and after the child's death.

c. Share your own memories and feelings with the sibling.

d. Use physical touch as a way of reassuring and comforting the sibling.

The Neonate with Altered Health Status

- Explain the etiology, prognosis, and patient outcomes of common disorders affecting the preterm newborn.
- Describe the pathophysiologic principles related to developmental alterations in the term newborn.
- Describe the nursing assessment measures that help to identify developmental disorders and common problems associated with the high-risk newborn.
- Identify appropriate uses of the Ballard scale, the neonatal behavioral assessment scale, and the assessment of the preterm newborn behavioral scale that assist the healthcare team in identifying developmental disorders and healthcare problems of high-risk newborns.
- Discuss nursing care for a neonate with altered health status.
- Identify interdisciplinary interventions commonly used for each health challenge in newborns.

SECTION I: ASSESSING YOUR UNDERSTANDING

Activity A *Match the term in column A with the description in column B.*

Column A

____ **1.** Perinatal asphyxia

____ **2.** Patent ductus arteriosus

____ **3.** Intraventricular hemorrhage

____ **4.** Necrotizing enterocolitis

____ **5.** Neonatal sepsis

Column B

a. Condition resulting from premature newborn's inability to adequately respond to infection

b. The most common brain injury occurring in premature infants

c. Persistence of a fetal shunt between the pulmonary artery and aorta

d. Condition resulting from bowel wall ischemia with subsequent bacterial invasion

e. Condition arising from any interruption in blood flow and oxygen delivery during birth

Activity B *Indicate whether the following statements are true or false.*

1. T F Clavicular fractures are the most common fractures diagnosed as birth trauma.

2. T F Damage to the central nervous system from intraventricular hemorrhage can be reversed.

3. T F Kangaroo care involves skin-to-skin holding.

4. T F   Radiant warmers decrease the amount of heat loss resulting from convection.

5. T F   Jaundice occurring within the first 24 hours of life is considered a normal finding.

Activity C *Fill in the blanks.*

1. The placenta allows glucose to cross from the mother to the fetus, but _____ does not cross.

2. Increased pressure on the fetus's head may cause _____ hemorrhages.

3. Necrotizing enterocolitis is initiated when the fetus shunts blood away from vital organs during _____, causing bowel ischemia.

4. The specific manifestation of traits, known as _____, produces the observable characteristics of the person.

SECTION II: APPLYING YOUR KNOWLEDGE

Activity D *Consider the scenario and answer the questions.*

Regina, a premature infant born several days ago with Apgar scores of 5 at 1 minute and 6 at 5 minutes, received surfactant therapy via endotracheal tube and was placed on a ventilator. The nurse in the neonatal intensive care unit (NICU) on the day shift is preparing to care for her. Regina's axillary temperature is 96.1 °F (35.6 °C) and her heart rate 115 beats per minute. She is lying uncovered in an open isolette. Her skin appears mottled with acrocyanosis. Louise, Regina's mother, asks if she can bathe Regina because she hasn't been bathed in a few days.

1. Based on the assessment findings, what might be going on with Regina? Explain why Regina is at risk for this condition.

    _____

    _____

2. What nursing interventions would be appropriate to implement based on the assessment?

    _____

    _____

3. Should the nurse allow Louise to bathe Regina at this time? Why or why not?

    _____

    _____

SECTION III: PRACTICING FOR NCLEX

Activity E *Choose the best answer for each question.*

1. The nurse is providing support to the parents of a premature infant who weighs less than 1,000 g and has severe intraventricular hemorrhage (IVH). Which of the following approaches will be of most value to the parents' ability to cope?
    a. "Let me tell you about skin-to-skin care."
    b. "We're increasing oxygen and body intravenous fluids."
    c. "What do you know about intraventricular hemorrhage?"
    d. "You are welcome to be with your baby."

2. The nurse is educating the parents of a premature infant with surfactant deficiency. Which comment would be most appropriate in helping the parents understand this condition?
    a. "Your child has suffered hypoxemia."
    b. "The lungs need treatment with surfactant."
    c. "The danger of pneumothorax is passed."
    d. "Each breath is like blowing up a new balloon."

3. When providing developmental care for a sick neonate, which of the following would the nurse integrate into the plan of care?
    a. Adapting interventions based infant response
    b. Offering nipple feeding when the child fusses
    c. Keeping a set schedule of activities
    d. Following a similar routine for each newborn

4. The nurse is caring for a premature neonate born at 27 weeks. Which condition would most likely present the greatest challenge to ensuring adequate neonatal nutrition?
    a. Poor muscle tone
    b. High caloric requirements
    c. Periodic breathing
    d. Poor sucking reflex

5. A premature neonate with hyperbilirubinemia is receiving phototherapy that uses green lights. Which of the following would the nurse anticipate related to this type of lighting?

   a. Limitation of parental bonding opportunities

   b. Increase in metabolic rate

   c. Appearance of the child as sicker

   d. Increased risk of dehydration from watery stools

6. The nurse is assessing a preterm newborn for signs and symptoms of increased intracranial pressure. Which of the following would the nurse expect to find? Select all that apply.

   a. Sunken fontanel

   b. Widening sutures

   c. Apnea

   d. Increased lethargy

   e. Decreased head circumference

   f. Seizures

The Child with Altered Cardiovascular Status

Learning Objectives

- Identify genetic, environmental, maternal, and multifactorial influences on congenital heart disease.
- Describe specific assessment skills that assist in the identification and care of the child with altered cardiovascular status.
- Identify invasive and noninvasive diagnostic tools that help in evaluating children with suspected heart disease.
- Describe information to include in the teaching plan when preparing a pediatric cardiac patient for a procedure.
- List nursing interventions and potential complications during the acute and convalescent phases of postoperative care for the cardiac patient.
- Explain the pathophysiology associated with, presentation of, and interdisciplinary interventions for the child with heart failure, cyanosis, and acquired heart disease.
- Describe the anatomic variations associated with the more common congenital defects, and explain the hemodynamic consequences of these defects.
- Discuss the various medical and surgical treatments of congenital heart defects, and differentiate between curative and palliative procedures.

SECTION I: ASSESSING YOUR UNDERSTANDING

Activity A *Fill in the blanks.*

1. _____ is an acquired heart defect that is diagnosed by the Jones criteria.

2. _____ is an acquired heart defect that is given aspirin and intravenous immunoglobulin to reduce the risk of coronary artery abnormalities.

3. _____ are given to prevent an infection of the endocardial surface of the heart before dental procedures.

4. _____ involves the use of catheters threaded into the heart to visualize the anatomy of the heart chambers or blood vessels and assists in treating the child's condition.

5. _____ is a clinical syndrome in which the heart's pumping ability is inadequate to meet the metabolic demands of the body.

Activity B *Match the following clinical signs in column B with the type of Jones criteria in column A. You may use the answers more than once.*

Column A	Column B
____ **1.** Major manifestation	**a.** Carditis
	b. Polyarthritis
____ **2.** Minor manifestation	**c.** Chorea
	d. Fever
____ **3.** Acute phase	**e.** Increased ESR

Activity C *Write the correct pathophysiologic sequencing for a child in heart failure with left ventricular heart dysfunction.*

1. ventricles dilate

2. heart failure

3. LVEDP increases

4. Systemic engorgement

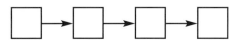

Activity D *Briefly answer the following.*

1. Name the potential environmental factors that may cause congenital heart defects.

   _____

   _____

   _____

2. What would the nurse be palpating for on the chest wall of a child with a congenital heart defect?

   _____

   _____

   _____

3. What is the purpose of percutaneous balloon angioplasty with regard to a pulmonary stenosis?

   _____

   _____

   _____

4. What nursing interventions would the nurse perform on an infant with tetralogy of Fallot who becomes cyanotic?

   _____

   _____

   _____

5. What is the difference between primary and secondary hypertension?

   _____

   _____

   _____

SECTION II: APPLYING YOUR KNOWLEDGE

Activity E *Consider the scenario and answer the questions.*

Sally is a 1-week-old infant who is brought to the pediatrician's office for poor feeding and lethargy. Sally was a full-term infant, vaginal delivery, with no complications during pregnancy or delivery. This is the parent's second child and they do not think Sally is acting like their first child did at this age. They remember their other child being much more vigorous. The parents state the poor feeding and lethargy really started more this morning. When the nurse is checking Sally in for her appointment, the following assessment findings were discovered: weight down 4 oz since birth; heart rate, 190 beats per minute; respiratory rate, 80 breaths per minute; and Sally appears cyanotic.

1. Based on this history and assessment findings, what types of interventions would the nurse perform?

   _____

   _____

2. What is the probable cause of this problem and what can the nurse anticipate will happen to the infant?

   _____

   _____

SECTION III: PRACTICING FOR NCLEX

Activity F *Briefly answer the questions.*

1. In fetal circulation, blood flows from the placenta through the _____ to the fetus.

2. _____ is the heart defect that can be characterized by decreased blood pressure in the lower extremities and increased blood pressure in the upper extremities.

3. _____ banding is used to decrease pulmonary blood flow to the lungs.

4. _____ medications include dopamine, dobutamine, milrinone, and epinephrine.

Activity G *Choose the best answer.*

1. An 8-year-old child is in the hospital for gastroenteritis, and a heart murmur is noticed. The doctor has ordered an echocardiogram. How would the nurse educate the parents about this?
   a. "All children with heart murmurs get an echocardiogram."
   b. "Heart murmurs could be a sign of a congenital heart defect."
   c. "This is a test to measure the impulses of the heart."
   d. "Your child is too old to have a congenital heart defect, but this test will show if there has been damage to the heart."

2. A child with Down syndrome also has a congenital heart defect. What education should be provided to the parents about children with Down syndrome and the cause of heart defects?
   a. "Heart defects are commonly associated with Down syndrome."
   b. "The heart defect was probably caused by environmental factors."
   c. "Heart defects occur related to medication the mother was taking while pregnant."
   d. "The echocardiogram will tell us what caused the heart defect."

3. A parent brings an infant in for an evaluation at the pediatrician's office. Which of the following symptoms would indicate a possible cardiac defect in an infant?
   a. Vertigo
   b. Poor feeding
   c. Chest pain
   d. Rash

4. A parent is in the office with her 2-month-old for a checkup. What would be included in a cardiovascular assessment of the infant?
   a. Range of motion testing
   b. Newborn reflexes
   c. Head circumference
   d. Respiratory rate

5. A child with a congenital heart defect is getting a cardiac catheterization. How would this test be described to the parent by the nurse?
   a. "This is a test that will check how blood if flowing through the heart."
   b. "This is a test that will check the electrical impulses in the heart."
   c. "This test can only determine the size of the heart."
   d. "This is an invasive test that can also provide an intervention of the heart if needed."

6. A 5-year-old is getting a cardiac catheterization. What would be included prior to the procedure?
   a. Have the child meet a person dressed in a catheterization uniform.
   b. Give acetaminophen prior to the procedure if the child has a fever.
   c. Place an IV line in the foot for easy access.
   d. After the child is sedated, elevate the head of the bed.

7. Palliative surgery is being performed on a child with a hypoplastic left heart. What is the best explanation of this procedure to the parents?
   a. "The surgery will allow the child's condition to become more stable."
   b. "This type of procedure may cure the heart defect."
   c. "This is the only surgery your child will need for the heart defect."
   d. "The surgery will be exploratory in nature."

8. A nurse explains to the parent that the infant will need continuous blood pressure monitoring after heart surgery. How would the nurse explain the way in which this will be done?
   a. "This is performed through a cuff placed on the infant's leg."
   b. "This is monitored through the peripheral IV."
   c. "This is monitored by the central IV."
   d. "This is performed by probes placed on the infant's chest wall."

9. A nurse is administering albumin to a child who just had heart surgery. What is the rationale for administering albumin?
    a. It will increase fluid volume
    b. It is used as an intravascular volume expander
    c. It is a vasodilator to reduce afterload
    d. It is an inotropic medication to maintain cardiac output

10. The nurse is noticing peripheral vasoconstriction, assessed as cold feet and poor capillary refill time postoperatively of a child with a heart defect. This can be an early sign of which of the following?
    a. Decreased cardiac output
    b. Respiratory distress
    c. Allergy to medication
    d. A normal reaction after surgery

The Child with Altered Respiratory Status

Learning Objectives

- Describe the developmental and biologic variances in children's respiratory systems that predispose them to respiratory problems.
- Describe the common alterations in health patterns within the respiratory system in children in terms of etiology, pathophysiology, clinical manifestations, and interdisciplinary interventions.
- Describe the nursing assessment of the child with compromised respiratory function.
- Discuss the nursing care responsibilities associated with diagnosis of respiratory difficulties in children.
- Select the treatments that are most effective for specific respiratory conditions.
- Select nursing care interventions to support the child with an acute or chronic respiratory illness.

SECTION I: ASSESSING YOUR UNDERSTANDING

Activity A *Match the term in column A with the description from column B.*

Column A

____ **1.** Allergic rhinitis

____ **2.** Sinusitis

____ **3.** Bronchiolitis

____ **4.** Cystic fibrosis

____ **5.** Bronchopulmonary dysplasia

____ **6.** Asthma

____ **7.** Bronchitis

____ **8.** Croup

Column B

a. Clinical syndrome of hoarseness, inspiratory stridor, a "croupy" or barking cough, and varying degrees of respiratory distress

b. Transient inflammatory process involving the distal trachea and major bronchi

c. Chronic lung disease of children that begins in infancy

d. Autosomal recessive genetic condition that affects multiple systems

e. Chronic inflammatory disorders of the airways involving marked hyper-responsiveness

f. Condition characterized by sneezing; nasal itching; thin, watery rhinorrhea; and nasal congestion

g. Acute inflammation and obstruction of the bronchioles generally occurring during the first 2 years of life

h. Viral or bacterial infection in which complications such as orbital cellulitis can occur as a result of local extension of the disease

Activity B *Indicate whether the following statements are true or false.*

1. **T F** A child's airway is smaller in diameter but longer in length than an adult's airway.

2. **T F** Children with respiratory problems may exhibit retractions that increase the work of breathing.

3. **T F** Respiratory failure occurs when the arterial oxygen tension decreases to less than 80 mm Hg.

4. **T F** Stridor is a harsh, grating, whistling sound resulting from turbulent airflow through an obstruction.

5. **T F** Before suctioning a tracheostomy, the nurse should instill saline to thin the secretions.

Activity C *Fill in the blanks.*

1. The infant with Pierre Robin syndrome must be maintained in the _____ position as much as possible.

2. The child with allergic rhinitis typically has _____ rhinorrhea.

3. The paranasal sinuses include the _____, _____, _____, and _____ sinuses.

4. Tonsillitis most commonly affects _____ children.

5. _____ is the cessation of airflow in to and out of the lungs.

SECTION II: APPLYING YOUR KNOWLEDGE

Activity D *Consider the scenario and answer the questions.*

Carmella Ronzoni brings her 6-year-old son, Dominic, to the clinic. Dominic has been sneezing and has a clear, watery nasal discharge. Carmella states, "I think he has a cold, but I want to make sure. He always seems to get these same symptoms this time of the year." Assessment reveals bilateral nasal congestion and reddened, swollen nasal mucosa. Dominic tells the nurse that his eyes feel itchy and they are watery, but denies any sore throat. Dominic is afebrile. Allergic rhinitis is suspected.

1. What findings would help the nurse to differentiate whether Dominic was experiencing allergic rhinitis or a cold? What additional information would the nurse need to collect?

_____

_____

2. What medications might the healthcare provider prescribe for Dominic?

_____

_____

3. What teaching would be necessary for Carmella and Dominic related to allergic rhinitis?

_____

_____

SECTION III: PRACTICING FOR NCLEX

Activity E *Choose the best answer.*

1. A child is brought to the emergency department by his parents. The child is exhibiting respiratory distress. Which finding would the nurse interpret as most important?
   a. Wheezing
   b. Retractions
   c. Grunting
   d. Vesicular breath sounds

2. Which of the following would be the focus of care for an infant with choanal atresia?
   a. Maintaining airway patency
   b. Providing adequate nutrition
   c. Promoting optimal weight gain
   d. Educating the parents

3. A child with a history of recurrent throat infections is diagnosed with acute tonsillitis, and a decision is made to schedule the child for an outpatient tonsillectomy and adenoidectomy. The nurse informs the parents that the surgery will most likely be scheduled at which time?
   a. Within the next week
   b. Within 2 to 3 weeks
   c. One month from now
   d. In approximately 3 months

4. After teaching a group of students about croup syndromes, the instructor determines that additional teaching is needed when the students identify which of the following as an example?

   a. Acute epiglottis

   b. Laryngotracheobronchitis

   c. Bacterial tracheitis

   d. Bronchiolitis

5. The nurse instructs the parents of a child with influenza to avoid aspirin products because of the increased risk for which of the following?

   a. Foreign body obstruction

   b. Apnea

   c. Reye syndrome

   d. Bacterial meningitis

6. Which of the following instructions would be most appropriate to give to the parents of a child with bronchitis?

   a. "Allow the child to remain as active as possible."

   b. "Use cough suppressants."

   c. "Avoid exposing the child to irritants."

   d. "Limit the amount of fluids given to the child."

7. When describing asthma to a local group of parents, which of the following would the nurse include?

   a. "Asthma accounts for a small amount of pediatric hospitalizations."

   b. "It is the leading cause of school absenteeism resulting from a chronic condition."

   c. "The prevalence of asthma is highest in Hispanics."

   d. "The condition involves irreversible changes in the airway."

CHAPTER 17

The Child with Altered Fluid and Electrolyte Status

Learning Objectives

- Discuss the physiologic principles that regulate fluid and electrolyte balance.
- Compare total water distribution, intracellular fluid, and extracellular fluid in infants, children, and adults.
- Review assessment parameters for a child at risk for fluid or electrolyte imbalance.
- Identify laboratory tests used to assess fluid and electrolyte balance.
- Calculate maintenance fluid therapy requirements and identify nursing care priorities for a child receiving intravenous fluid therapy.
- Discuss nursing care measures for the child receiving parenteral nutrition.
- Describe the assessment and treatment of hypertonic and hypotonic dehydration.
- Explain the principles of acid–base balance.
- Discuss the causes and treatment of specific electrolyte imbalances.

SECTION I: ASSESSING YOUR UNDERSTANDING

Activity A *Fill in the blanks.*

1. _____ is the type of electrolyte imbalance characterized by a serum sodium level less than 130 mEq/L.

2. _____ is the type of electrolyte imbalance characterized by a serum sodium level more than 150 mEq/L.

3. _____ is the type of electrolyte imbalance characterized by a serum potassium level less than 3.5 mEq/L.

4. _____ is the type of electrolyte imbalance characterized by inadequate phosphorus intake, particularly prevalent in preterm infants who have high phosphorus needs because of rapid growth.

5. _____ is the type of electrolyte imbalance that can be caused by excessive intake of vitamin D. Parents should be instructed to keep vitamin supplements out of children's reach and tell them about the hazards of excessive vitamin supplementation.

Activity B *Match the following signs of dehydration with the appropriate level of dehydration. You may use the answers more than once.*

Column A

____ 1. Mild dehydration

____ 2. Moderate dehydration

____ 3. Severe dehydration

Column B

a. Normal blood pressure and dry mucous membranes

b. Lethargic and non-palpable pulse

c. Sunken fontanel and tenting of the skin

d. Restless and 8% weight loss

e. Low urine output and 5% weight loss

63

Activity C *Put in order the signs of dehydration from mild to severe in terms of changes in heart rate.*

1. _____

2. _____

3. _____

Activity D *Briefly answer the following.*

1. Describe the purpose of the arterial blood gases test.

   _____

   _____

   _____

2. Describe the purpose of the urine specific gravity test.

   _____

   _____

   _____

3. Describe what may cause stool color changes.

   _____

   _____

   _____

4. Describe the nursing interventions associated with hypophosphatemia.

   _____

   _____

   _____

5. Describe the nursing interventions associated with hypercalcemia.

   _____

   _____

   _____

SECTION II: APPLYING YOUR KNOWLEDGE

Activity E *Consider the scenario and answer the questions.*

Jamie is a 2-year-old who has been vomiting for the past 16 hours. He has not urinated in 12 hours and is appearing lethargic, so Jamie is brought to the pediatric office for an evaluation. When the nurse is "triaging" Jamie, the following is noted: weight, 22 lb; temperature, 37 °C; lips, dry; Jamie is crying at times and not producing tears; heart rate, 160 beats per minute with a weak, thready pulse; respiratory rate, 30 breaths per minute; skin temperature, cool. Jamie's previous weight was 24 lb 2 months earlier. Jamie's mother has been giving him milk to try to keep him hydrated because that is the "only thing he will drink." The main question the mother wants to know is if there is anything that can be given to stop Jamie's vomiting.

Upon examination by the nurse practitioner, a diagnosis of acute gastroenteritis is made. It is determined that Jamie is dehydrated and will need treatment for that.

1. Describe what type of dehydration Jamie is experiencing and describe the symptoms in the scenario that helped you make this decision.

   _____

   _____

2. What type of educational information would be given to the parent?

   _____

   _____

SECTION III: PRACTICING FOR NCLEX

Activity F *Fill in the blanks.*

1. _____ is the type of electrolyte imbalance with a serum magnesium level exceeding 2.3 mEq/L.

2. _____ is the type of electrolyte imbalance characterized by a serum magnesium level less than 1.5 mEq/L.

3. _____ is the type of electrolyte imbalance characterized by a total calcium level exceeding 10.8 mEq/L.

4. _____ is the type of electrolyte imbalance whose most serious manifestations can cause cardiovascular changes.

5. Before administering _____, ensure that the child is producing urine, which demonstrates renal function.

Activity G *Choose the best answer.*

1. A nurse is concerned an asymptomatic child may become dehydrated because he has been having diarrhea. Which of the following nursing interventions would be appropriate?

   a. The nurse should not perform any intervention.

   b. The nurse would administer IV fluids.

   c. The nurse would perform teaching about dehydration.

   d. The nurse should administer antidiarrheal medication.

2. A parent asks how his child can lose fluids if she is are not vomiting. What is the best response by the nurse?

   a. "Fluids can be lost through sweating and breathing as well."

   b. "Fluids are only lost in urine."

   c. "Fluids are lost through saliva."

   d. "Fluids are mainly lost from blood draws."

3. A parent asks how her infant can be dehydrated if he did not even seem thirsty for the formula. What is the best response by the nurse?

   a. "If the bottle was offered, the infant would have taken it."

   b. "The infant was not thirsty."

   c. "The infant must have not have been dehydrated then."

   d. "The infant's thirst mechanism is not fully developed."

4. A nurse is assessing a child's fluid and electrolyte status. What is an important aspect of assessment of this area?

   a. All body systems should be included in the assessment.

   b. The assessment should mainly focus on kidney function.

   c. The assessment should mainly focus on skin integument.

   d. All body systems except for a neurologic examination would be included.

5. A parent asks why his child is experiencing decreased alertness if she is just dehydrated. What is the best response by the nurse?

   a. "The child is just tired from being sick."

   b. "The child is, more than likely, in pain."

   c. "The child's neurologic system is affected with dehydration."

   d. "The child's respiratory system is affected and causes decreased oxygen."

6. A child who is dehydrated is experiencing decreased blood pressure. The nurse is concerned about this for which of the following reasons?

   a. Decreased blood pressure is a late sign of fluid volume deficit.

   b. This is the child's normal way of compensating for fluid loss.

   c. This is the body's way of increasing output.

   d. Decreased blood pressure is an early sign of fluid volume deficit.

7. When caring for a child that is dehydrated, which of the following would be a priority?

   a. Encourage the use of oral fluids.

   b. Immediately start an IV for fluid administration.

   c. Obtain intraosseous access for fluid administration.

   d. Obtain central venous access.

8. A nurse is caring for a child with a PICC line. Which of the following would be a complication the nurse would watch for with this type of line?

   a. Diarrhea

   b. Neurologic changes

   c. Abdominal perforation

   d. Fever

9. According to the nurse's calculations, a doctor is prescribing less than the amount of IV fluid than the drug book recommends for the child's weight. What is the most likely reason for this discrepancy?

   a. This is a mistake and the doctor should be notified.

   b. This is a result of the fact that the child has a renal impairment.

   c. This is the result of the fact that the child has a burn causing dehydration.

   d. It is important always to give less than the amount required.

10. A nurse tells the family the child is experiencing abnormal fluid losses. What is the potential cause of these losses?

    a. Increased respiratory rate

    b. Sweating

    c. Suctioning

    d. Fever

The Child with Altered Gastrointestinal Status

Learning Objectives

- Discuss components of the history and physical assessment that are important to consider when evaluating a child with an alteration in gastrointestinal status.
- Identify specific tests and laboratory results that assist the healthcare team in identifying alterations in gastrointestinal status.
- Discuss diet modifications and alternative feeding methods used to treat alterations in gastrointestinal status.
- Review the important pathophysiologic principles that help to differentiate gastrointestinal disorders.
- Describe the interdisciplinary interventions commonly used for disorders of the gastrointestinal system.

SECTION I: ASSESSING YOUR UNDERSTANDING

Activity A *Fill in the blanks.*

1. Proper function of the GI system is essential for normal growth and for maintaining

   _____ _____ _____
   balances.

2. _____ is the primary source of carbohydrate in breast milk and most infant formulas.

3. During the first 3 days of life, the infant has _____ stools that are dark-green/black, thick, and sticky.

4. A(n) _____ is a surgically created opening between the GI tract and the outside of the body.

5. _____ _____ is the gold standard for infant feeding.

6. _____ _____ _____ feedings are administered slowly over 12 to 24 hours and are used when feedings are being delivered into the small intestine.

7. _____ _____ results from incomplete or failed fusion of embryologic structures, the maxillary and medial nasal elevations, between the fifth and eighth weeks of gestation.

8. _____ _____ is a congenital defect that results in complete obstruction of the bowel.

Activity B *Match the blood study in column A with its purpose listed in column B.*

Column A	Column B
____ **1.** Assess for signs of bleeding	**a.** Bilirubin
	b. Platelet count
____ **2.** Determine protein synthesis and promote wound healing	**c.** Prothrombin time
	d. Fibrinogen
	e. Zinc
____ **3.** Monitor patients with severe liver failure	**f.** Ammonia
	g. Total protein, albumin

____ **4.** Evaluate efficacy of coagulation system

____ **5.** Assess for sepsis or liver disease

____ **6.** Monitor nutritional status and liver function

____ **7.** Determine forms of jaundice

Activity C *Place the following physical assessment techniques in the order in which they should be performed to obtain an accurate assessment of bowel sounds.*

1. Inspection

2. Percussion

3. Palpation

4. Auscultation

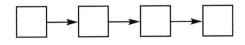

Activity D *Briefly answer the following.*

1. List the four primary functions of the gastrointestinal system.

_____

_____

_____

2. Describe three activities involved in the care of the child receiving enteral nutrition.

_____

_____

_____

3. Note three teaching points for the family of a young child being discharged with an enteral feeding tube.

_____

_____

_____

4. List four malformations of the upper GI tract that can affect GI function.

_____

_____

_____

5. Briefly describe two inflammatory disorders of the GI tract.

_____

_____

_____

6. Describe three possible causes of idiopathic acute pancreatitis.

_____

_____

_____

7. List four disorders of GI motility and function.

_____

_____

_____

8. Give two interdisciplinary interventions used to treat functional abdominal pain or irritable bowel syndrome.

_____

_____

_____

SECTION II: APPLYING YOUR KNOWLEDGE

Activity E *Consider the scenario and answer the questions.*

Ella, age 20, is a single mother of a 13-month-old baby boy named Jakob. Ella brings Jakob to the community healthcare clinic for a checkup. The nurse examining him notes that the infant appears apathetic and listless, and responds to physical stimulation by flinching and turning away from the stimulus. A physical assessment confirms that Jakob is below the normal expected growth standards, and his medical history states that Jakob has no underlying GI problems diagnosed that would be responsible for his failure to thrive.

Ella confides to the nurse that she is living with her mother and works as a waitress during the lunch shift. She also attends school part-time in the evenings to obtain her GED. Ella admits to being too exhausted to properly oversee Jakob's feeding schedule and leaves most of the care of Jakob to her mother. She further states that she "can't wait to graduate and get a good job," because her mother is tired of the responsibility of taking care of Jakob.

1. What information should the nurse share with Ella regarding Jakob's condition and what are the long-term effects that Jakob may suffer as a result of failure to thrive?

   _____

   _____

2. What nursing services might the nurse provide for this family that may ease the burden of care for Jakob and improve his prospects for living a normal life?

   _____

   _____

SECTION III: PRACTICING FOR NCLEX

Activity F *Choose the best answer.*

1. A pediatric nurse is performing a physical assessment of the gastrointestinal system of 7-year-old Jason. Jason flinches and cries when touched by the nurse. Which of the following interventions would be most helpful for calming Jason?
   a. Tell Jason he will get a lollipop if he is good during the examination.
   b. Demonstrate parts of the examination on a stuffed animal.
   c. Drape Jason to avoid unnecessary exposure.
   d. Keep the examination tools out of Jason's sight.

2. A nurse examines a 5-year-old boy brought to the emergency room by his mother. The mother tells the nurse that her son has been passing stool with red blood and a mucuslike substance. Based on this finding, what GI condition might the nurse suspect?

   a. Cystic fibrosis
   b. Biliary atresia
   c. Intussusception
   d. Anal fissures

3. Twelve-year-old Jeremy is brought to the health clinic by his parents. The parents tell the nurse that Jeremy has been vomiting bright-red blood. What type of condition might this indicate?
   a. Upper GI bleeding
   b. Lower GI bleeding
   c. GI obstruction
   d. Biliary tract obstruction

4. The nurse is preparing a diet for 10-year-old patient with esophageal stricture. Which one of the following is a recommended diet for this patient?
   a. High fiber
   b. High protein, high calorie
   c. Fat controlled
   d. Puree, mechanical, soft

5. The pediatric nurse is caring for a 5-year-old boy with an anorectal malformation classified as intermediate. Which of the following is one diagnosis that fits in this category?
   a. Anocutaneous fistula
   b. Rectobulbar urethral fistula
   c. Anorectal agenesis
   d. Rectal atresia

6. Parents of an 8-year-old diagnosed with gastroenteritis ask the nurse what could have caused the condition and if there are certain foods they should avoid in the future. The nurse's best response is as follows:
   a. "Gastroenteritis is caused by microorganisms that are not found in food products."
   b. "Unwashed fruits and vegetables are the most common causes of food-borne agents causing gastroenteritis."
   c. "Gastroenteritis is spread from person to person via a parasite; it is not caused by foods."
   d. "Certain types of fish may contain non-microbial agents that can cause gastroenteritis."

7. A nurse caring for a patient with Crohn's disease teaches a student nurse how to distinguish this disease from ulcerative colitis. Which of the following is an indicator for Crohn disease?
   a. Absence of fistulas or strictures
   b. Continuous, uniform lesions
   c. Shallow ulcerations limited to mucosal and submucosal layers
   d. Presence of granulomas

8. A mother brings her 2-year-old son to the health clinic. She tells the nurse that her son, who she is attempting to potty train, has not had a bowel movement in 3 days and she is worried about constipation. The nurse explains to the mother that there are many causes of constipation besides metabolic or structure disorders, including which of the following?
   a. A diet high in fiber
   b. Starting toilet training too late
   c. Excessive dairy intake
   d. Obesity

9. The nurse caring for patients with cirrhosis knows that the disease can be caused by many conditions, including which of the following?
   a. Cystic fibrosis
   b. Diabetes mellitus
   c. Hypothyroidism
   d. Myelomeningocele

10. The nurse performs tube care for a patient with an enteral feeding tube. Which of the following describes a recommended action for this type of care?
    a. Monitor position of the G tube or G-J tube before each feeding and with site care by pulling back gently on the tube to ensure position.
    b. If the tube becomes dislodged, disregard the tube and insert another tube.
    c. Flush the tube with saline after each intermittent feeding or every 4 to 6 hours during continuous feedings, per protocol.
    d. Administer medications in a crushed form, including enteric-coated and time-release medications.

Activity G *Choose all answers that apply.*

1. The nurse caring for neonates in the NICU reviews the medical conditions that contribute to organic failure to thrive. Which of the following GI conditions are responsible for this condition?
   a. Gastroesophageal reflux disease
   b. Pyloric stenosis
   c. Celiac disease
   d. Hirschsprung's disease
   e. Cerebral palsy
   f. Diabetes insipidus

2. The nurse is examining an infant with a suspected bowel obstruction. What tests might be ordered to confirm this diagnosis?
   a. Abdominal x-ray
   b. Barium swallow
   c. Upper gastrointestinal series
   d. Gastric emptying study
   e. Liver biliary scan
   f. Anorectal manometry

3. A nurse is caring for an 18-month-old female who is postoperative for surgery to correct a cleft palate. Which of the following are priority nursing interventions for this patient?
   a. Setting up a high humidity oxygen tent
   b. Observing the child for bleeding and excess mucus in the mouth
   c. Teaching the parents how to care for the incision at home
   d. Explaining to the parents the procedure performed and how to care for the child at home
   e. Administering pain medication as prescribed
   f. Positioning the child on her abdomen with the head of the bed elevated 30 degrees

The Child with Altered Genitourinary Status

Learning Objectives

- Correlate the child's history, symptoms, and physical signs with manifestations of genitourinary abnormalities.
- Identify various diagnostic procedures and their applications in genitourinary evaluation.
- Describe the treatment options available to children with alterations in genitourinary status.
- Describe common alterations in health patterns related to the genitourinary system.
- Identify the teaching needs of the child experiencing challenges related to urinary elimination.
- Describe the types of renal replacement therapies available for the child experiencing acute renal failure or chronic renal disease.
- Choose nursing interventions that support the interdisciplinary plan of care for the child with a genitourinary disorder.

SECTION I: ASSESSING YOUR UNDERSTANDING

Activity A *Fill in the blanks.*

1. _____ therapies include peritoneal dialysis, hemodialysis, and kidney transplant.

2. _____occurs in young girls experiencing symptoms of burning, dysuria, frequency, or vaginal itching. They may have a UTI, but more commonly, the symptoms are caused by irritation of the skin at the opening of the urethra or around the vaginal area.

3. _____ is a type of enuresis during which the child achieves continence for at least 6 months but then resumes incontinence.

4. _____ is a derivative of ADH and reduces the volume of urine produced during sleep for control of nocturnal enuresis.

5. _____ is a congenital anomaly of the penis in which the urethral folds fail to fuse in the midline, and the urethral meatus opens on the ventral surface of the penis.

Activity B *Match the following the types of disorders in column A with the most likely clinical signs in column B. You may use the answers only once.*

Column A

_____ 1. Nephrotic syndrome

_____ 2. Glomerulone-phritis

_____ 3. Hemolytic ure-mic syndrome

_____ 4. UTI

_____ 5. Testicular torsion

Column B

a. Proteinuria and hematuria

b. Bloody diarrhea and purpura

c. Fever and dysuria

d. Associated with the bell clapper deformity

e. Associated with a recent strep throat infection

Activity C *Starting with grade 2, describe each grade in the order of what occurs in VUR.*

_____

_____

_____

Activity D *Briefly answer the following.*

1. Describe the function of the kidneys in utero up until 2 years old.

   _____

   _____

   _____

2. Describe how a kidney donor is matched to a recipient.

   _____

   _____

   _____

3. Describe the difference between primary and secondary enuresis.

   _____

   _____

   _____

4. Describe techniques that would facilitate examination of the testicles.

   _____

   _____

   _____

5. Describe paraphimosis.

   _____

   _____

   _____

6. What would be included in teaching a parent about a first UTI in their 3-yearold daughter?

   _____

   _____

   _____

SECTION II: APPLYING YOUR KNOWLEDGE

Activity E *Consider the scenario and answer the questions.*

The nurse is performing an admission history on a male adolescent who is being admitted for asthma. All pertinent information about the current admission is obtained and the nurse begins asking a review of systems assessment. When the teen is asked about the genitourinary system, he states he is having a heavy feeling in his testicle. He thinks he may have coughed too hard with his asthma and is worried he may have a hernia. He has also been sexually active and does not want his parents to know, so he did not say anything to them about the feeling in his testicle.

1. A "bag of worms" feeling was noted on examination of the left testicle. Based on these findings, what would be the appropriate education to provide to the teen?

   _____

   _____

2. What information should be given to the teen about the treatment of this problem?

   _____

   _____

SECTION III: PRACTICING FOR NCLEX

Activity F *Fill in the blanks.*

1. _____ is a condition in which urine backs up into the renal pelvis and calyces, which dilate and impair renal function.

2. Short _____ in females younger than 5 years old are a common cause of UTIs.

3. _____ catheters should be avoided because of the increased chance of an allergic reaction.

4. _____ removes waste products and corrects serum chemistry values of the child's blood by circulating it through an extracorporeal circuit.

5. _____ occurs if the urinary tract infection extends to the kidneys.

Activity G *Choose the best answer.*

1. A nurse is instructing a parent to obtain a first-morning urine sample. Which of the following would be included in the education?

   a. The urine should be kept in the refrigerator.

   b. The urine should be kept at room temperature.

   c. The urine should be collected by a catheter at the hospital.

   d. The urine should be collected by a catheter at home by the parent.

2. A child is having a stoma placed to divert the urine out of the bladder through the skin. The nurse would explain that this is what type of stoma?

   a. Ureterostomy

   b. Pyelostomy

   c. Vesicostomy

   d. Double-J stent

3. A parent is asking when his child will be ready to complete his own self-care of intermittent catheterization. What is the best response by the nurse?

   a. "The child is usually ready between 6 to 8 years old."

   b. "The child is usually ready by 5 years old."

   c. "The child is usually ready between 8 to 10 years old."

   d. "The child is usually ready by 12 years old."

4. A child is having catheter function problems during dialysis. Which of the following would the nurse know is a potential cause of the catheter problem?

   a. Constipation

   b. Diarrhea

   c. Fever

   d. Cold symptoms

5. When teaching a parent about clean intermittent catheterization, which of the following would be included in the education?

   a. Sterile gloves should be worn during the procedure.

   b. This is considered a clean procedure.

   c. This should be performed two times daily.

   d. This should be performed as needed for bladder distension.

6. Knowing the causes of morbidity with peritoneal dialysis, which of the following signs and symptoms would be important for the nurse to observe for?

   a. Abdominal pain

   b. Tachycardia

   c. Bradycardia

   d. Hematuria

7. When providing teaching to parents of a child who recently had an arteriovenous fistula placed, which of the following would be included to check for patency?

   a. The parent should check for a bruit daily.

   b. Once-a-month appointments for patency checks are important.

   c. The parent should check for a thrill once a week.

   d. Once a month, the parent should check for a thrill.

8. A parent wants to know the purpose of HLA (human lymphocyte antigen) typing. What is the best response by the nurse?

   a. "This process examines the white blood cells to check for antibodies."

   b. "This process examines the red blood cells to check for compatibility."

   c. "This process examines the platelets for antibodies."

   d. "This process examines the white blood cells for compatibility."

9. A parent is asking for information about what to expect after her child gets a kidney transplant. What information would the nurse give to the parent?

   a. "The child can stop the transplant medication after surgery."

   b. "The child needs to continue taking anti-rejection medication after surgery."

   c. "Antirejection medications will need to be taken by IV for 3 months after surgery."

   d. "Immunosuppressant medications may be stopped after 1 year."

10. Which of the following would be a potential complication if cystitis is left untreated?

    a. Hypertension

    b. Hydronephrosis

    c. VUR

    d. *Escherichia coli*

20

The Child with Altered Musculoskeletal Status

Learning Objectives

- Recognize clinical signs and symptoms that would indicate a musculoskeletal disorder or injury.
- State the interdisciplinary interventions that are commonly used for each musculoskeletal disorder or injury.
- Explain nursing care interventions to promote healing and prevent further injury and skin breakdown in the child receiving treatment for a musculoskeletal disorder or injury.
- Provide family education regarding home care, activity, and dietary modifications for the child with a musculoskeletal disorder or injury.
- Describe measures to protect children from musculoskeletal injury.

SECTION I: ASSESSING YOUR UNDERSTANDING

Activity A *Fill in the blanks.*

1. Teenagers undergoing treatment for scoliosis often prefer a _____ brace because it is not visible when worn under clothing.

2. _____ is used to turn the child who has undergone spinal fusion.

3. The term *luxation* refers to frank dislocation; _____ is partial dislocation.

4. Most experts believe that if a spinal curve reaches _____ degrees or more, surgery should be considered because there is a great possibility that the curve will worsen.

5. *Kyphosis* and _____ are two terms used to describe a spinal curvature in the sagittal plane.

6. Much of the skeleton in an infant or young child consists of preosseous cartilage and growth plates called _____.

7. _____ is an infection of the bone and the tissues around the bone.

Activity B *Match the term in column A with the proper definition in column B.*

Column A	Column B
___ 1. Fasciotomy	a. Surgical incision made through fascia
___ 2. Reduction	b. Insufficient bone tissue
___ 3. Osteopenia	c. Restore proper anatomic alignment
___ 4. Antalgic	d. Immobility and consolidation of joints
___ 5. Ankylosis	e. Limping on affected side

Activity C *Match the type of sprain in column A with the descriptive phrase in column B.*

Column A	Column B
___ 1. First-degree sprain	a. Ligament is completely torn and joint is unstable
___ 2. Second-degree sprain	b. Ligament is stretched and affected joint is stable

_____ **3.** Third-degree sprain

c. Ligament is partially torn and joint laxity is noted on examination

Activity D *Place the following steps in the proper sequence.*

1. The pathophysiology of healing for a fractured bone:

  a. Osteoblast activation

  b. Remodeling

  c. Inflammation

  d. Callus formation

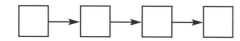

2. The common sites for septic arthritis in decreasing order of prevalence:

  a. Ankles

  b. Wrists

  c. Elbows

  d. Pelvis

  e. Shoulders

  f. Hips

  g. Knees

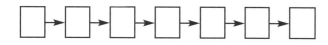

Activity E *Briefly answer the following.*

1. Briefly describe the three types of traction.

_____

_____

_____

2. Explain how to differentiate metatarsus adductus from clubfoot.

_____

_____

_____

3. State the reason why osteomyelitis requires immediate treatment if suspected.

_____

_____

_____

4. Describe the classic sign of compartment syndrome.

_____

_____

_____

SECTION II: APPLYING YOUR KNOWLEDGE

Activity F *Consider the scenario and answer the questions.*

Anita has recently given birth to a baby with developmental dysplasia of the hip (DDH). She is very anxious about her newborn's diagnosis and is asking a number of questions regarding treatment, therapy, and short- and long-term complications. Anita is concerned that she did something during her pregnancy to cause this defect.

1. As the nurse caring for Anita and her baby, what information would you share with her to alleviate her fears regarding her causing this condition in her newborn?

_____

_____

2. What are the priority assessments the nurse should perform? Does the child's age influence the assessment and assessment findings?

_____

_____

3. The newborn is going to be placed in a spica cast, followed by a Pavlik harness. Develop a discharge teaching plan for Anita and her child.

_____

_____

SECTION III: PRACTICING FOR NCLEX

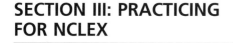 *Choose the best answer.*

1. Syndrome of inappropriate antidiuretic hormone (SIADH) is common in spinal fusion patients after surgery. Which of the following is usually the first indicator of SIADH?

    a. Increase in urine output

    b. Decrease in urine output

    c. Decrease in blood pressure

    d. Increase in respiratory rate

2. The nurse is caring for a 12-year-old boy who has recently been diagnosed with scoliosis. He is very upset about the prospect of wearing a brace and is dismayed because he believes it is a "girl's disease." Which of the following would best address this boy's concerns?

    a. "If you wear your brace properly, you may not need surgery."

    b. "Let's talk to a boy who wears a brace and is on a swim team."

    c. "The good news is boys usually have less progression than girls."

    d. "Let's talk to the doctor about your treatment options."

3. A 6-year-old boy has been diagnosed with septic arthritis of the hip and is now ready for discharge from the hospital. The parents feel extremely guilty about not seeking medical attention earlier. Which of the following discharge instructions would be most helpful to the parents and ensure proper home care?

    a. Prepare a written medication schedule and remind the parents to finish the medication prescribed even if the child feels better.

    b. Suggest ways to increase the child's daily fluid and fiber intake to prevent possible constipation.

    c. Teach the parents how to assess and record their child's temperature and pain level daily.

    d. Emphasize keeping the child's follow-up appointments with the physician because the development of osteomyelitis is possible.

4. The nurse is caring for a 10-year-old girl who has recently been diagnosed with juvenile arthritis. She is experiencing discomfort and generalized body stiffness in the mornings before school. The girl is one of four school-aged children in the family, and her mother is seeking guidance on helpful ways to overcome this early-morning stiffness. Which of the following suggestions would be most appropriate in this situation?

    a. Taking a warm bath every morning as soon as she awakens

    b. Paraffin baths for her hands would relieve stiffness

    c. Using an electric blanket an hour before she awakens

    d. Sleeping on a waterbed would likely ease stiffness

5. The nurse is caring for a 13-year-old girl with systemic lupus erythematosus (SLE) who is on steroid therapy. The girl is upset about her weight gain, particularly in her face, and is becoming resistant to taking her medicine. Which of the following comments will be the most helpful?

    a. "You need to take your medicine every day or you might trigger an acute episode."

    b. "Weight gain is a common side effect of steroid treatment, as is your facial fullness."

    c. "Here is a pamphlet so that you can read about the treatment of your disease."

    d. "Let's put you in touch with some other girls who are on the same medicine for SLE."

6. The nurse is caring for an 18-month-old child with a fracture of the left humerus, and abuse is suspected. The physician orders an x-ray. Which of the following findings could rule out abuse and indicate osteogenesis imperfecta (OI)?

    a. Multiple fractures in long bones

    b. Lack of swelling at the fracture site

    c. Bruising of the affected arm

    d. Spiral fracture of the humerus

7. Parents have sought evaluation of their 5-year-old child because he is pigeon-toed and trips over his feet when he runs. He has been diagnosed with femoral anteversion. The parents are panicking because the doctor mentioned surgery is necessary in approximately 1% of the cases to correct the anteversion. Which of the following would best address their concerns?
   a. "Remember, less than 1% of children actually need surgery."
   b. "This condition usually resolves spontaneously by age 9."
   c. "Surgery would not be considered until a few years from now."
   d. "The recovery from surgery for his condition takes only about 6 weeks."

8. A 12-year-old boy is being treated for Legg-Calve-Perthes disease (LCPD) and requires traction. His mother is divorced and works full-time. She is skeptical about the seriousness of her son's condition because he appears so healthy. She is resistant to the plan for home traction. Which of the following would be most helpful to initiate treatment and ensure compliance?
   a. "Without traction, your son could develop permanent mobility difficulties."
   b. "There are community resources to help with your son's treatment and care."
   c. "We can easily teach you the principles of traction and immobilization."
   d. "We can make arrangements with the school for home tutoring."

9. A nurse is watching her son's soccer game. One of the other players falls to the ground with an injury to his foot. He is in extreme pain and cannot bear weight on his foot. The coach is transporting the boy to the emergency room and seeks the advice of the nurse before they leave. Which of the following is the most important instruction?
   a. Take off his shoe
   b. Leave his shoe in place
   c. Apply ice to his foot
   d. Elevate his foot above his heart

10. The nurse is assisting a 9-year-old girl who is waiting for her physician to apply a fiberglass cast to her wrist. The girl is very nervous and is afraid that the process will be painful. Which of the following would provide support to the girl?
    a. "Don't worry; it will only take a few minutes."
    b. "The cast doesn't hurt going on or when they take it off."
    c. "The cast will stabilize your wrist and help it heal."
    d. "Would you like to choose the color of your cast?"

Activity H *Choose all answers that apply.*

1. A nurse performing a physical assessment of a 10-year-old documents the following nursing diagnosis: Impaired physical mobility related to use of leg brace. Which of the following nursing interventions would be appropriate for this patient? (Choose all that apply.)
   a. Encourage the child to participate in all care decisions for the brace.
   b. Use serial manipulation to restore joint mobility.
   c. Assess the patient for signs of skin breakdown.
   d. Encourage early return to weight-bearing activity.
   e. Assist the child to perform ROM exercises four times daily.
   f. Allow the child to perform tasks at his own rate.

2. The nurse caring for children with musculoskeletal conditions is aware that the following diagnostic tests can be used to detect infection. (Choose all that apply.)
   a. CBC (complete blood count)
   b. CRP (C-reactive protein)
   c. Calcium and phosphorous levels
   d. Erythrocyte sedimentation rate
   e. Blood culture and sensitivity
   f. Arthrography

3. The nurse assists in fluid aspiration from the joints of a 12-year-old patient experiencing swollen ankles. Which of the following conditions might this test diagnose? (Choose all that apply.)
   a. Bone tumor
   b. Traumatic arthritis
   c. Fracture
   d. Synovial abnormalities
   e. Systemic lupus erythematosus
   f. Rheumatoid arthritis

4. A nurse helps plan a healthy diet high in phosphorous for a patient diagnosed with rickets. Which of the following phosphorous rich foods might be included? (Choose all that apply.)
   a. Egg yolks
   b. Tomatoes
   c. Green vegetables
   d. Whole-grain cereals
   e. Legumes
   f. Citrus fruits

5. Henry is a 13-year-old diagnosed with a Salter-Harris classification of type II epiphyseal fracture. The nurse caring for Henry knows that the characteristics of this classification of fracture include which of the following? (Choose all that apply.)
   a. It may be mistaken for a sprain
   b. It does not usually affect growth
   c. There is a fracture separation of the epiphysis
   d. Open reduction and internal fixation are usually necessary
   e. It results in premature closure of the epiphyseal plate
   f. Circulation remains intact

The Child with Altered Neurologic Status

Learning Objectives

- Identify components of the neurologic assessment.
- Examine the effect of embryonic development on the child's neurologic functioning.
- Explain the purposes of diagnostic tests used in the assessment of the child with altered neurologic status.
- Discuss the treatment modalities that can be selected to therapeutically manage the needs of the child with altered neurologic status.
- Identify common neurologic conditions that children may experience, and their causes and defining characteristics.

SECTION I: ASSESSING YOUR UNDERSTANDING

Activity A *Fill in the blanks.*

1. Nerve cells use the process of _____ to develop connections with each other.

2. The surgeon creates a flap opening of the skull during a _____ procedure.

3. Complications from altered responsiveness and immobility can create risk of the _____ syndrome.

4. Altered neurologic status creates potential for long-term _____ affecting cognitive and motor functioning.

5. _____ is the mechanism by which brain matter, blood, and CSF alter their volumes to maintain normal intracranial pressure.

6. Bulging fontanels may indicate increased intracranial pressure; sunken fontanels may indicate _____.

7. Characteristic body positions, called _____ and decerebrate posturing, indicate brain dysfunction.

Activity B *Match the headache type in column A with the proper etiology in column b.*

Column A

___ 1. Migraine

___ 2. Tension

___ 3. Traumatic

___ 4. Rebound

___ 5. Infectious

___ 6. Structural disorder

Column B

a. Head or neck injury

b. Increased ICP

c. Neuronal process

d. Muscular/emotional

e. Substance use/ withdrawal

f. Intracranial infection

Activity C *Match characteristics in column I with either breath holding (column A) or seizure (column B) by placing a mark in the appropriate column.*

Column I: Characteristic	Column A: Breath Holding	Column B: Seizure
1. Onset 6 to 18 months of age	☐	☐
2. Rarely precipitating event	☐	☐
3. Crying at onset	☐	☐
4. Cyanosis	☐	☐
5. Typically convulsions	☐	☐

6. Incontinence ☐ ☐
7. Unconscious ☐ ☐
8. Postictal confusion ☐ ☐
9. Bradycardia ☐ ☐
10. Abnormal EEG ☐ ☐

Activity D *Place the following in the proper order.*

1. Forms of assessment for an emergency situation:
   a. Acute neurologic check
   b. Brief screening examination
   c. Comprehensive neurologic assessment

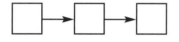

2. Developmental events:
   a. Myelination
   b. Neuronal proliferation
   c. Neural tube formation
   d. Synaptogenesis

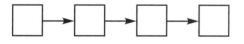

Activity E *Briefly answer the following.*

1. Describe the elements that compose a comprehensive neurologic assessment.

_____

_____

_____

2. Note the primary elements of nursing care for a child with increased ICP.

_____

_____

_____

3. Describe nursing care for a child who has a head injury.

_____

_____

_____

4. List the primary aspects of postoperative nursing care for a child with spina bifida.

_____

_____

_____

5. Describe the major components of the health history and physical examination for the child with signs and symptoms of hydrocephalus.

_____

_____

_____

SECTION II: APPLYING YOUR KNOWLEDGE

Activity F *Consider the scenario and answer the questions.*

Paul, age 17, is brought to the emergency room in an ambulance after a motor vehicle accident in which he was the sole occupant of the car. Paul sustained a serious head injury and shows signs of intracranial swelling, with an ICP of 47 mm Hg. He lost consciousness after the injury and is still unconscious upon admittance to the emergency room. After an examination, his physician orders a craniotomy to drain collecting blood from the skull. Paul's parents anxiously stand by their son with looks of fear on their face. The mother vocally blames herself for allowing her son, who just recently received his driver's license, to drive to work on his own. The father asks what is involved in a craniotomy and if the operation will cause any permanent damage to their son's brain. He questions whether the procedure is necessary and asks the nurse what would happen if they did not consent to the surgery.

1. What would be the nurse's best response to the mother's question?

_____

_____

2. What psychosocial nursing skills would the nurse use to prepare the client and family for the surgery?

_____

_____

3. What nursing care would the client require pre- and postoperatively?

_____

_____

SECTION III: PRACTICING FOR NCLEX

Activity G *Choose the best answer.*

1. The nurse is caring for a 9-month-old who has undergone surgery to correct the effects of craniosynostosis. Which of the following nursing interventions is most important to perform at this stage?

   a. Show the parents before-and-after photos

   b. Put elbow splints on the child

   c. Explain the use of the hard-shell helmet

   d. Notify the physician if the child's eyes swell shut

2. The nurse is caring for a 6-year-old child with meningitis. Which of the following interventions would be effective for this child?

   a. Manage reduced fluid intake

   b. Take droplet precautions for 7 to 14 days

   c. Administer analgesics to eliminate pain

   d. Start IV antibiotics after CSF culture results

3. A 9-year-old child with brain abscesses resulting from an untreated, abscessed tooth is under the nurse's care. Which of the following interventions is appropriate for managing the child's condition?

   a. Manage care based on results of lumbar puncture

   b. Take droplet precautions prior to IV antibiotics

   c. Educate parents about IV administration

   d. Monitor to avoid respiratory distress

4. The nurse is taking a health history for a 10-year-old boy who is experiencing difficulty swallowing and stiffness in his jaw. Which of the following responses from the child and parent would suggest the child has tetanus?

   a. The child has been vomiting frequently

   b. The mother says he had a DT shot 2 years ago

   c. The child cut his hand with a kitchen knife

   d. The child cut his finger while camping a week ago

5. The nurse is caring for a 6-year-old child with Guillain-Barré syndrome. Which of the following activities would be most valuable in managing this disorder?

   a. Preparing the parents for the loss of the child

   b. Monitoring for change in intracranial pressure

   c. Moving the child's arms and legs periodically

   d. Showing parents how to administer IV antibiotics

6. A 10-year-old boy received a mild concussion and seems normal. His parents are anxious to get him out of the hospital. What is the best example of family teaching regarding the care of this patient?

   a. "Bring him back if he has any problems related to the injury."

   b. "Be patient. There are a number of things you need to know."

   c. "What's your hurry? Do you know how serious head injuries are?"

   d. "He's going to be just fine. You can take him home now."

7. The nurse is caring for a male newborn with a slightly enlarged head. Which of the following interventions should be used?

   a. Educate the mother about changes in head size

   b. Measure head circumference and plot growth

   c. Find out what the mother knows about hydrocephalus

   d. Pinch the child to see if he responds

8. The nurse is caring for a 9-year-old with a head injury. Which of the following interventions is most effective for this client?

   a. Monitor to prevent fluid overload

   b. Show parents how to use diazepam rectally

   c. Support parents when they grieve

   d. Let the child listen to his favorite music

9. A 2-year-old had a mild seizure subsequent to a fever. Which of the following nursing actions will be most appropriate?

   a. Assure the parents that the seizures are benign

   b. Advise that the child will not need to undergo further diagnostic testing

   c. Show parents how to use diazepam to prevent seizures

   d. Inform parents that recurrent seizures will not require treatment

10. The nurse is caring for a 16-year-old boy with bacterial meningitis. Which of the following would be most important in educating this client about the disorder?

   a. "You got in here just in time. This could have killed you!"

   b. "We have to stop the inflammation to the covering of your brain."

   c. "This spreads by mouth and nose droplets during close contact."

   d. "You're going to have a headache until we get your temperature down."

Activity H *Choose all answers that apply.*

1. The pediatric nurse is caring for a 6-year-old patient with cerebral edema. Which of the following interventions would the nurse perform to limit secondary cerebral injury from brain tissue swelling?

   a. Allow ICP to return to baseline between nursing activities

   b. Increase stimuli in patient's environment

   c. Administer anticonvulsants, as appropriate

   d. Position patient with head of bed slightly lowered

   e. Push fluids

   f. Perform passive range-of-motion exercises

2. Which of the following assessments/interventions are appropriate for a patient after cranial surgery?

   a. Monitor for Cushing's triad and report it immediately

   b. Maintain neutral position of head and neck

   c. Avoid palpating infant fontanels

   d. Administer extra fluids to maintain hydration

   e. Give daily antidiarrhea medication

   f. Encourage deep-breathing exercises

3. A pediatric nurse is discharging a patient who was placed under observation after an epileptic seizure. Which of the following appropriately describes family teaching to mange a child during a seizure that should be included in the discharge plan?

   a. After seizure, do not hyperextend the neck

   b. Allow seizures to end without interference

   c. Remove child's eyeglasses to prevent injury to the face

   d. Wrap the child in a tightly secured blanket during seizures

   e. Place a tongue depressor wrapped in gauze in the child's mouth

   f. After the seizure, place the child in a supine position with the head in a midline position

4. The nurse caring for a 12-year-old who is experiencing a myasthenic crisis is aware that the following symptoms distinguish this condition from cholinergic crisis.

   a. Anoxia

   b. Cyanosis

   c. Increased urinary output

   d. Anticholinergic drug toxicity

   e. Bowel and bladder incontinence

   f. Absence of swallow reflex and cough

The Child with a Malignancy

CHAPTER **22**

Learning Objectives

- Identify abnormal findings that can be identified by physical assessment of a child with a malignancy.
- Describe the nursing care for children undergoing diagnostic tests to detect and diagnose pediatric malignancies.
- Describe the treatment modalities used for children with malignancies.
- Describe the interdisciplinary interventions to minimize the treatment-related side effects associated with each type of malignancy.
- Identify the psychosocial needs of children with malignancies and their families.
- Differentiate the types of malignancies commonly found in the pediatric population.

SECTION I: ASSESSING YOUR UNDERSTANDING

Activity A *Fill in the blanks.*

1. _____ is the second leading cause of death in children, exceeded only by accidents.

2. _____ therapy is accomplished by providing various combinations of therapies, such as multiagent chemotherapy, radiation, surgery, hematopoietic stem cell transplantation, and biologic response modifiers.

3. _____ _____ is the most common tumor that precedes both hematologic and nonhematologic secondary tumors.

4. A child is considered to be a cancer survivor when he or she has been disease free for _____ years past the end of the maintenance phase of chemotherapy.

5. _____ therapy is cytotoxic by damaging the synthesis of nucleic acids, causing breaks in the DNA or RNA molecule, or causing double-stranded breaks in the molecules.

Activity B *Match terms associated with cancer chemotherapy in column A with the definition listed in column B.*

Column A

____ 1. Induction

____ 2. Relapse

____ 3. Remission

____ 4. Observation phase

____ 5. Maintenance phase

Column B

a. A temporary or permanent response to therapy that causes a decrease or absence of the primary malignancy

b. The initial phase of chemotherapy

c. Phase of chemotherapy when treatment is finished

d. Cancer returns

e. Designated period during which treatment is continued to destroy any residual cancer cells

Activity C *Place the following stages of chemotherapy in the order in which they are initiated in the process.*

1. Maintenance

2. Induction

3. Remission

4. Observation

5. Consolidation

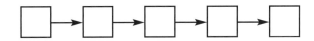

Activity D *Briefly answer the following.*

1. Describe how cancers in children differ from cancers in adults.

   _____

   _____

   _____

2. List two factors that cause signs and symptoms of cancer in children.

   _____

   _____

   _____

3. Give the characteristics of a stage III rhabdomyosarcoma.

   _____

   _____

   _____

4. Note three nursing responsibilities for the child receiving radiation treatments.

   _____

   _____

   _____

5. List two mechanisms of action of biologic response modifiers (BRMs).

   _____

   _____

   _____

6. Give three stressors related to the family receiving a diagnosis of cancer for a family member.

   _____

   _____

   _____

SECTION II: APPLYING YOUR KNOWLEDGE

Activity E *Consider the scenario and answer the questions.*

Megan is a 9-year-old who has been brought to the free community clinic by her father, John. John tells the nurse that Megan has been overly tired lately and has not had a good appetite for more than a week. Upon examination, Megan appears pale and thin with lymph nodes that are firm and painful on palpation. The physician orders a chest x-ray to check for cancer. John tells the nurse that he is a single father who recently lost his job and is living on workman's compensation. He further states that he is worried about whether he will be able to afford treatment for Megan or care for her if she is sick.

1. What type of cancer is usually indicated by Megan's symptoms?

   _____

   _____

2. What nursing interventions could the nurse use to support Megan and her father during diagnostic testing?

   _____

   _____

3. If there is a diagnosis of cancer, what psychosocial skills might the nurse use to help this family prepare emotionally and financially for the necessary treatments and care?

   _____

   _____

SECTION III: PRACTICING FOR NCLEX

Activity F *Choose the best answer.*

1. A nurse examining 3-year-old Kayla observes asymmetry of her facial features. What cancerous condition might this symptom indicate?
   a. Retinoblastoma
   b. Soft-tissue sarcoma
   c. Hodgkin's disease
   d. Bone tumor

2. The nurse examining 9-year-old Nathan documents the presence of pallor, ecchymoses, and petechiae. The physician orders a complete blood count. Nathan's mother asks the nurse why the physician is ordering a blood test. What is the nurse's best response?
   a. "Nathan is displaying the signs and symptoms of Hodgkin's disease, which is diagnosed by a blood test."
   b. "The signs Nathan is displaying are indicative of a soft-tissue sarcoma and a blood count will confirm this diagnosis."
   c. "With the presence of pallor, ecchymoses, and petechiae, we have to rule out a blood disorder, such as leukemia."
   d. "Don't be overly worried about the blood test for leukemia; 90% of the time these tests are negative."

3. A nurse is assisting with a lumbar puncture for a 7-year-old patient. Which of the following is a recommended measure to prepare the child for this test?
   a. Withhold fluids before the procedure
   b. Empty the bladder before the procedure
   c. Push fluids after the procedure
   d. Use clean technique for the procedure

4. A pediatric patient's CBC with differential test shows increased WBC with the presence of lymphoblasts. The nurse knows that this may indicate which of the following?
   a. Neutropenia
   b. Anemia
   c. Thrombocytopenia
   d. Leukemia

5. The nurse notices that the CBC test of a patient suggests malfunctioning bone marrow. Which test will commonly be performed next to examine the cell type and morphology?
   a. Bone marrow aspiration and biopsy
   b. Serum chemistries
   c. Absolute neutrophil count
   d. Urine catecholamine VMA, HVA

6. The nurse examines 5-year-old Penny, who is exhibiting bruising around her eyes (proptosis). What type of malignancy may cause this condition?
   a. Anemia
   b. Soft-tissue mass
   c. Lymphadenopathy
   d. Retinoblastoma

7. Marisa is a 16-year-old who has leukemia. Her parents ask the nurse what they can do to help their adolescent through the recovery process. Which of the following is the nurse's best response to this question?
   a. "Make sure Marisa rests over the summer by limiting her usual activities."
   b. "Allow Marisa to tell her school peers about her condition herself."
   c. "Plan to have Marisa back in school as soon as possible after her illness."
   d. "Encourage Marisa to be dependent on nurses and family for physical care."

8. Leroy is an 8-year-old diagnosed with Burkitt's lymphoma. The nurse caring for Leroy knows that this cancer has a primal occurrence in which location?
   a. Cranium
   b. Abdomen
   c. Liver
   d. Lungs

9. A patient presents with the following characteristic triad of signs and symptoms: paresis of conjugate gaze, pyramidal tract involvement, and cerebellar pathway signs. The nurse knows these signs are indicative of which of the following?
   a. Medulloblastoma
   b. Cerebral astrocytoma
   c. Ependymoma
   d. Brain stem glioma

10. A pediatric nurse caring for children with cancer recognizes the signs and symptoms of tumor lysis syndrome in a patient. Which one of the following is an appropriate intervention for this emergency condition?

   a. Provide IV hydration to flush cell by-products through the kidneys

   b. Administer broad-spectrum antibiotics

   c. Provide blood product transfusions

   d. Initiate emergency radiation or steroids to reduce tumor mass

Activity G *Choose all answers that apply.*

1. The nurse caring for patients with cancer knows that the following are characteristics of child cancer that differ from adult cancer.

   a. Child cancers are more common than adult cancers.

   b. Child cancers involve tissue.

   c. Child cancers are usually nonepithelial.

   d. Child cancers have a long period from initiation to diagnosis.

   e. Child cancers have a strong relationship to environmental exposures.

   f. Child cancers are very responsive to chemotherapy.

2. A nurse recognizes the signs of septic shock in a 6-year-old patient with Hodgkin's disease. These symptoms include which of the following?

   a. Tachycardia

   b. Tachypnea

   c. Peripheral vasodilation

   d. Leukocytosis

   e. Uncontrolled bleeding

   f. Diminished or absent bowel sounds

3. A 19-year-old patient diagnosed with an infratentorial brain tumor exhibits the following common signs of this disease documented by the nurse. (Choose all that apply.)

   a. Increased intracranial pressure

   b. Headaches

   c. Ataxia

   d. Seizures

   e. Abnormal reflexes

   f. Personality changes

Activity H *Fill in the blanks.*

1. The nurse caring for a child scheduled for a hematopoietic stem cell transplantation (HSCT) explains to the parents that the stem cells for HSCT are obtained from _____ _____ or from _____ or _____ blood.

2. The nurse assisting with stem cell transplantation knows that two kinds of transplants are performed: _____, which uses the child's own stem cells, and _____, which uses a matched donor's stem cells.

Alterations in Hematologic Status

- Describe how assessment data are used to identify and manage bleeding disorders, hemoglobinopathies, and anemias in children.
- Discuss the role of the healthcare team in preparing children and families for various diagnostic studies that help to identify and manage hematologic disorders.
- Summarize the interventions by the healthcare team during transfusion therapy.
- Discuss the rationale for the interdisciplinary interventions used in managing pediatric hematologic alterations.
- Describe the nursing care of children with bleeding disorders, hemoglobinopathies, and anemias.

SECTION I: ASSESSING YOUR UNDERSTANDING

ACTIVITY A *Fill in the blanks.*

1. The hematologic system is responsible for transporting _____ _____ to, and _____ _____ from, cells throughout the body.

2. The hematologic system plays a crucial role in _____ (blood clotting), immunity, and heat regulation.

3. The _____ _____ is the earliest stage in the development of all blood cells.

4. People living in high-altitude environments generally produce a greater number of red blood cells and develop physiologic _____ (an excess of red blood cells).

5. When bleeding occurs, healthcare interventions focus on managing the bleeding promptly. Areas of bleeding are revealed by ecchymoses, epistaxis (nosebleeds), _____ (blood in the urine), _____ (vomiting blood), and _____ (bloody stool, also called *melena*).

6. The production and maturation of red blood cells is affected by nutritional intake of _____, vitamin B_{12}, and _____ _____.

7. The _____ _____ leads to formation of a red thrombus or clot in response to an abnormality in the vessel wall in the absence of tissue injury.

8. A disorder in hemostasis is called a(n) _____.

Activity B *Match the disorders of hemostasis listed in column A with their definitions in column B.*

Column A

____ 1. Sickle cell disease

Column B

a. Characterized by a lack of precursor cells for the platelets, red blood cells, and white blood cells that are

____ 2. Disseminated intravascular coagulation

____ 3. Hemophilia

____ 4. Hemarthrosis

____ 5. Acquired aplastic anemia

____ 6. Hereditary spherocytosis

____ 7. Thrombocytopenia

____ 8. Von Willebrand disease

____ 9. Idiopathic thrombocytopenic purpura

____ 10. Thalassemia

normally present in the peripheral circulation

b. Most common hereditary bleeding disorder

c. Characterized by a decrease or absence of one or more of the normal globin chains in the hemoglobin molecule and by ineffective erythropoiesis

d. Serious bleeding disorder caused by decreased, absent, or dysfunctional procoagulant factor

e. An abnormally low concentration of circulating platelets

f. Abnormalities in the beta globin chains of the hemoglobin molecule

g. An acquired, self-limiting disorder of hemostasis characterized by destruction and decreased numbers of circulating platelets

h. Acquired coagulopathy characterized by thrombosis and hemorrhage

i. Deep bleeding into joints

j. Characterized by loss of surface area on the red blood cell membrane

Activity C *Place the following in their proper order of occurrence.*

1. Hematologic system developmental events:

   a. Liver shows evidence of hematopoiesis

   b. Blood islands evident in yolk sac

   c. Blood formation occurs

d. Bone marrow becomes involved in blood cell production

e. Circulation is evident

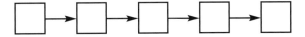

2. Developmental order of organs according to their production of white blood cells:

   a. Thymus

   b. Lymph nodes

   c. Liver

   d. Spleen

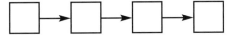

3. White blood cells according to their sequential development as the myeloid lineage:

   a. Macrophages

   b. Monoblasts

   c. Monocytes

   d. Myeloblasts

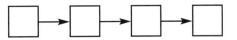

Activity D *Briefly answer the questions.*

1. List the two reasons that hematopoiesis depends on the stem cell.

_____

_____

_____

2. Describe how the erythrocyte (red blood cell) undergoes several developmental changes as it progresses through the prenatal period to infancy and childhood.

_____

_____

_____

3. Give three examples of common types of crisis events associated with sickle cell disease.

_____

_____

_____

4. Describe four teaching interventions for the child with iron deficiency anemia.

_____

_____

_____

5. List three factors that may precipitate sickling of red blood cells.

_____

_____

_____

6. Give three goals of a chronic transfusion therapy program for children with severe chronic anemia.

_____

_____

_____

SECTION II: APPLYING YOUR KNOWLEDGE

Activity E _Consider the scenario and answer the questions._

Jabir is a 10-year-old boy of African descent who was diagnosed with sickle cell disease as a baby. He is an only child, and his parents both have the sickle cell trait, but not the disease. They bring Jabir to the clinic for a checkup after an episode of pneumonia that required hospitalization a month earlier. He has also had two mild vasoocclusive crises during the past 3 years that were treated at home.

The nurse performing a physical assessment notes slight growth developmental delays and benign vascular changes in his eyes. Although Jabir appears healthy at this visit, the nurse collects baseline data to help manage future crises. Lab tests are ordered to assess hematologic status, liver function, and renal function.

In the past, Jabir's health condition did not appreciably interfere with the family's everyday routine or Jabir's active school life. However, in light of the recent hospitalization, Jabir's parents express their wishes to the nurse to become more proactive with their son's condition to prevent future crises.

1. How might the nurse direct the management of Jabir's sickle cell disease to optimize healthy outcomes?

_____

_____

2. What teaching interventions would be appropriate for Jabir and his family?

_____

_____

SECTION III: PRACTICING FOR NCLEX

Activity F _Choose the bet answer._

1. The nurse caring for a child with sickle cell disease knows that this condition is associated with an excess of which of the following?
   a. Hemoglobin F
   b. Hemoglobin C
   c. Hemoglobin B
   d. Hemoglobin A2

2. Jeremy is a 5-year-old diagnosed with neutropenia. The nurse caring for him is aware that which of the following is a sign of the disease?
   a. Bronchitis
   b. Thrush
   c. Tachycardia
   d. Enlarged spleen

3. A nurse performs a focused physical assessment on a 12-year-old patient who presents with tachypnea and sinusitis. A CBC with differential shows decreased platelet numbers indicative of which of the following?
   a. Anemia
   b. Pneumonia
   c. Thrombocytopenia
   d. Neutropenia

4. What test would be ordered for a neonate to detect hemolytic disease?
   a. Factor assays
   b. Hemoglobin electrophoresis
   c. Peripheral blood smear
   d. Coombs' test

5. The nurse performing testing on patients to evaluate hematologic status knows that the responsibilities of the nurse when performing total iron binding capacity (TIBC) and transferrin include which of the following?

   a. Ensuring that the child is fasting in the morning

   b. Placing the collected specimen on ice

   c. Performing the procedure using aseptic technique

   d. Protecting the sample from light

6. The nurse caring for a child with altered hematologic status assesses the child's tissue perfusion to indicate which of the following?

   a. Fluid balance

   b. Blood volume depletion

   c. Reduced oxygen carrying capacity of blood

   d. Infection

7. The nurse preparing a child for a transfusion reviews the measures used to prevent transfusion reactions, including which of the following?

   a. Priming the infusion line with normal saline to decrease the risk of hemolysis of red blood cells

   b. Administering the infusion quickly during the first 15 minutes of infusion

   c. Remaining with the child during the first 5 minutes of the transfusion

   d. Watching for transfusion reactions that typically occur within the first 10 minutes of administration

8. A nursing plan of care for a child with altered hematologic status should include which of the following interventions?

   a. Delay pain medication until the patient asks for it

   b. Encourage child to progress from passive ROM to active exercise

   c. Provide enemas for constipation to avoid Valsalva maneuver

   d. Give the child ibuprofen for pain

9. A nurse planning meals for a child diagnosed with anemia includes which of the following food that is high in iron?

   a. Whole grains

   b. Dried fruit

   c. Citrus fruit

   d. Eggs

10. The nurse assisting with a blood transfusion for a patient uses a fresh-frozen plasma product (FFP). This product is used for which of the following?

    a. Symptomatic anemia

    b. Replacement therapy

    c. Bleeding associated with thrombocytopenia

    d. Replacement of noncellular coagulation factors

11. A 6-year-old with sickle cell anemia receiving a blood transfusion displays symptoms of fever, urticaria, headache, hypotension, and shock. These are signs of which type of reaction?

    a. Febrile

    b. Allergic

    c. Hemolytic

    d. Overload

Activity G *Choose all answers that apply.*

1. The nurse performing a focused physical assessment contributes important information for determining hematologic disorders in patients. Which of the following accurately describes alterations and their clinical significance?

   a. Fever may be present with infections related to neutropenia

   b. Fatigue, pallor, and weight gain are common signs of anemia

   c. Bleeding, bruising, and petechiae are signs of thrombocytopenia

   d. Jaundiced sclera may be present with hemolytic anemia

   e. Dactylitis is a common sign of hemophilia

   f. Lower extremity ulcers may be an indication of anemia

2. The nurse caring for patients with sickle cell anemia explains to parents that which of the following are complications of the disease?
   a. Skin ulcerations
   b. Vascular changes in the eyes
   c. Decreased cardiac output
   d. Low liver enzyme levels
   e. Hyposthenuria
   f. Chronic lung disease

3. A patient with sickle cell disease is experiencing an acute splenic sequestration. The nurse knows that which of the following are symptoms of this type of crisis?
   a. Left upper quadrant abdominal pain and vomiting
   b. Presence of nucleated red blood cells
   c. Decreased platelet count
   d. Increased hemoglobin
   e. Increased hematocrit
   f. Decreased reticulocyte count

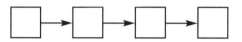 **Activity H** *Place the following events in the order in which hemostasis occurs after the loss of vascular integrity.*
   a. Formation of platelet plug
   b. Vasoconstrictive response
   c. Release of fibrin degradation products
   d. Formation of fibrin mesh

☐ → ☐ → ☐ → ☐

The Child with an Infectious Disease

- Discuss interventions that disrupt the chain of infection.
- Identify assessment findings specific to pediatric infections and the diagnostic criteria used to confirm diagnoses.
- Discuss nursing interventions to prevent the transmission of disease-causing organisms.
- Name the diseases that constitute the TORCH syndrome and describe the nursing care for congenitally infected infants.
- Compare the different herpes viruses and discuss the nursing care for each.
- Describe at least one key intervention to decrease the risk of transmission of human immuno-deficiency virus from a pregnant female to her fetus.
- Identify the symptoms of at least three tick-borne fevers and teaching needed to reduce transmission of tick-borne fevers.
- Name two sexually transmitted diseases and interventions to prevent transmission.
- Identify two infectious diseases that should be reported to the local health department for follow-up contact tracing.

SECTION I: ASSESSING YOUR UNDERSTANDING

Activity A *Briefly answer the following.*

1. Name the three most common tick-borne infections.

   _____

   _____

   _____

2. Describe the three phases of pertussis and the associated findings.

   _____

   _____

   _____

3. Explain how cytomegalovirus is transmitted.

   _____

   _____

   _____

4. Identify the triad of symptoms associated with mononucleosis.

   _____

   _____

   _____

5. Describe the two types of streptococci that cause disease.

_____

_____

_____

Activity B *Fill in the blanks.*

1. Children receive _____ immunity from their mothers transplacentally or through breast milk.

2. Disease-producing microorganisms are often called _____ agents.

3. _____ is also called *whooping cough.*

4. Epstein-Barr virus is the causative agent in _____.

5. Koplik spots are the hallmark finding of _____.

SECTION II: APPLYING YOUR KNOWLEDGE

Activity C *Consider the scenario and answer the questions.*

Eileen and Kevin Waters bring their 8-year-old daughter, Chelsea, to the clinic because she has developed a rash on her lower leg. Her father states, "It started out as a tiny red lump but now it has gotten bigger. The center of the rash seems to be fading and going away." When questioned, Chelsea says that she has a headache and feels tired. Further assessment reveals that Chelsea and her father were camping and hiking in the woods about 2 weeks ago as part of a Girl Scout activity. Lyme disease is suspected.

1. What additional questions would the nurse need to ask to help in determining Chelsea's condition?

_____

_____

2. If Lyme disease is diagnosed, what medication(s) would be prescribed most likely?

_____

_____

3. What information would the nurse include in a teaching plan for this family?

_____

_____

SECTION III: PRACTICING FOR NCLEX

Activity D *Choose the best answer.*

1. A child diagnosed with pertussis is in the paroxysmal phase. Which of the following would the nurse expect to assess?
   a. Runny nose
   b. Violent coughing
   c. Scratchy throat
   d. Clearing of the throat

2. A child develops community-acquired methicillin-resistant *Staphylococcus aureus* (MRSA) infection. Which of the following agents would the nurse expect the healthcare provider to prescribe?
   a. Vancomycin
   b. Oxacillin
   c. Erythromycin
   d. Trimethoprim–sulfasoxazole

3. When describing the infections caused by group B streptococcus, which of the following would the nurse include?
   a. Impetigo
   b. Meningitis
   c. Necrotizing fasciitis
   d. Pharyngitis

4. After teaching a group of students about mononucleosis, the instructor determines that the students need additional information when they identify which of the following as a common assessment finding?
   a. Sore throat
   b. Fever
   c. Lymphadenopathy
   d. Jaundice

5. An infant who is hospitalized develops roseola. Which intervention would be least appropriate?

  a. Instituting isolation precautions for the infant

  b. Following standard precautions

  c. Giving prescribed acetaminophen for fever

  d. Monitoring for febrile seizures

6. A nurse is preparing a presentation about measles for a group of parents with preschoolers and early school-aged children. Which of the following would the nurse include in the presentation?

  a. Outbreaks are common during the fall and summer

  b. Coughing or sneezing are means for spreading the disease

  c. Children are contagious about a week before the rash occurs

  d. The typical illness lasts about 3 to 4 days.

7. An adolescent is diagnosed with *Chlamydia* infection and is receiving treatment. The nurse understands that the adolescent will most likely receive treatment for which other sexually transmitted infection?

  a. Syphilis

  b. Genital herpes

  c. Gonorrhea

  d. Hepatitis B

25

The Child with Altered Skin Integrity

Learning Objectives

- Identify characteristics of the child's skin that make the child especially susceptible to injury.
- Perform a health history and physical examination that include a complete evaluation of the skin, hair, and nails.
- Select nursing diagnoses that articulate the needs of the child, family, and community for the child who has a skin condition.
- Describe the presenting signs and symptoms of skin conditions frequently seen in the pediatric population.
- Use strategies to prevent further spread of a skin condition or further damage to tissue that has altered skin integrity.
- Discuss therapies that are effective in treating conditions of the skin.

SECTION I: ASSESSING YOUR UNDERSTANDING

Activity A *Fill in the blanks.*

1. The amount and distribution of _____ in the epidermis account for the color of a person's skin.

2. The diagnosis of erythema toxicum neonatorium involves microscopic examination of scrapings from the pustules, which are stained with Wright's solution. If ETN is present, large numbers of _____ are detected.

3. _____ is frequently called *cradle cap* in infants or dandruff in older children.

4. Pubic lice are most commonly transmitted through intimate bodily contact, although they also may be transferred by _____, which are contaminated objects such as combs, brushes, and clothing.

5. Impetigo contagiosa is primarily caused by _____ and _____ organisms.

6. Warts are common, harmless skin growths (small epidermal tumors of the skin) caused by a _____.

7. A classic sign of _____ is the presence of a beefy, red, glazed, weeping dermatitis in the genital area.

8. _____ _____ occur in children and adolescents whose mobility, activity, or sensory perception is severely restricted because of prolonged immobilization or conditions that may impede movement.

9. _____, a saplike oil, produces an intense dermatologic inflammatory reaction upon contact with the skin.

10. When the urticaria extends deep into the dermis (subcutaneous or submucosal layers), it is known as _____ and is usually characterized by a tingling burning sensation in normal-appearing skin with overlying swelling.

Activity B *Match the types of dermatitis in column A with their cause in column B.*

Column A

____ **1.** Diaper rash

____ **2.** Contact

____ **3.** Atopic

____ **4.** Seborrheic

Column B

a. Overproduction of sebum

b. Exaggerated inflammatory response to environmental triggers

c. Prolonged contact with an irritant plus a diaper

d. Irritating or allergic substance

Activity C *Write the correct sequence in the boxes provided.*

1. The progression in a typical staphylococcal scalded skin syndrome (SSSS) case:

   a. Bullae enlarge and rupture to reveal a moist erythematous base. This process gives rise to the classic scalded appearance.

   b. The child develops fever, malaise, and extremely tender erythematous patches on the face, neck, axilla, and perineum.

   c. The child complains of a sore throat or conjunctivitis.

   d. Flaccid bullae develop within the erythematous areas.

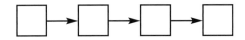

2. A typical hand, foot, and mouth disease case:

   a. Spread of the virus to the lymph nodes

   b. Appearance of lesions on the oral mucosa

   c. Extension of the disease to other secondary infection sites

   d. Virus implantation on the mucosa of the throat and ileum

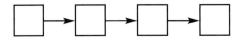

Activity D *Briefly answer the following.*

1. Name and describe the three primary treatment interventions for candidiasis.

_____

_____

_____

2. Name and describe the four stages of pressure ulcers.

_____

_____

_____

SECTION II: APPLYING YOUR KNOWLEDGE

Activity E *Consider the scenario and answer the questions.*

Jordan is a 10-year-old boy who was involved in a house fire. He was brought to the emergency department with burns on both of his hands and arms, his back, and half of his chest.

1. What percentage of his body was burned in the fire?

_____

_____

2. What are 3 nursing diagnoses that would be appropriate for this patient?

_____

_____

3. List the complications from burns that you would observe for.

_____

_____

SECTION III: PRACTICING FOR NCLEX

Activity F *Choose the best answer.*

1. A new African American mother brings her 2-week-old infant in for a regular checkup. She states to the nurse that she is very concerned about the bruising on her newborn's bottom. "I think he was injured during the delivery and the bruising just isn't getting any better." What would be the nurse's correct response?
   a. "Did you have a difficult delivery? Sometimes newborn's skin can bruise during a traumatic delivery. The bruises will fade over time."
   b. "The darker skin color you see on your newborn's bottom is a mongolian spot. It may fade some over time. It is a benign skin pigmentation."
   c. "The darker pigmentation you see can be an early sign of skin cancer. Your newborn should be taken to see a dermatologist as soon as possible."
   d. "Have you seen anyone handle your newborn in a rough manner? These spots can be an early sign of physical abuse."
2. Which of the following is true of erythema toxicum neonatorium?
   a. Cultures of the lesions are sterile
   b. Fever is often associated with it
   c. Poor feeding is a common symptom
   d. Lethargy can be expected
3. When educating the parents of a 4-year-old girl with severe psoriasis, the nurse should include which of the following as goals of therapy?
   a. Limit contact with other children
   b. Complete recovery
   c. Promote good nutrition
   d. Promote acceptance of the child's condition
4. When caring for a 15-year-old boy with acne vulgaris, which of the following is the best advice to give to him?
   a. "Avoid foods containing high amounts of fat and/or chocolate."
   b. "Take prescribed oral antibiotics at the same time every day."
   c. "Use a powerful astringent as part of your daily skin care regimen."
   d. "Pop each pimple with a clean needle just before it comes to a head."
5. The school nurse has just completed a periodic classroom check for lice and discovers nits on 9-year-old Lisa. The nurse phones Lisa's mom to pick her up from school. What is the most important instruction for the nurse to give to Lisa's mom?
   a. "All household animals must be treated as well."
   b. "Follow the written instructions on over-the-counter products containing lindane precisely."
   c. "Washing affected hair with dog shampoo, kerosine, or vinegar can be effective home remedies."
   d. "The more product used on the scalp, the more effective it is at killing the lice."
6. Stacy is a 10-year-old girl who has just been diagnosed with human papilloma virus, or genital warts. Which further assessment of this child would be most important for the nurse to perform?
   a. Sexual abuse
   b. Daily hygiene routines
   c. Treatments used at home
   d. Type of undergarments used by the child
7. Which of the following assessments is most important for the nurse to perform after the diagnosis of a fungal skin infection?
   a. Immunizations
   b. Daily hygiene routine
   c. Nutrition
   d. Respiratory

8. Which of the following is the best intervention for a child with a fungal skin infection?

   a. Remove all scales on the affected area daily

   b. Cleanse skin thoroughly before application of topical medications

   c. Apply oils or petroleum jelly to the infected skin and/or scalp

   d. Keep feet covered before, during, and after all sports

9. What is the best nursing care related to pressure ulcers?

   a. Reposition the child every 2 hours

   b. Keep skin dry and clean

   c. Prevention

   d. Use convoluted foam and gel pillows

10. When an adverse drug reaction is suspected, what is the first action that should be taken?

    a. Immediately stop administering the suspected drug

    b. Apply cortisone to the affected area

    c. Encourage fluid intake

    d. Apply a medical alert bracelet to the patient's wrist

11. What is the initial intervention done for a patient if carbon monoxide poisoning from a fire is suspected?

    a. Intubate the patient immediately

    b. Place an oxygen saturation probe on the patient

    c. Administer high concentrations of oxygen by mask until the condition is resolved

    d. Position the patient in semi–Fowler's position

12. The mother of 6-year-old girl believes her daughter may have contracted scabies after being exposed to it at school. Which of the following health history items is most valuable when determining if the mother is correct?

    a. The itching is primarily on the scalp

    b. The child has circular lesions with red borders

    c. The child uses only her own comb and brush

    d. The child is scratching her scalp mostly at night

13. The nurse is teaching the parents of a 3-year-old girl with hand, foot, and mouth disease how to care for her at home. Which of the following statements is the best choice for the nurse to make?

    a. "Keep her away from your pets at home."

    b. "She will have to stay home from day care for 3 weeks."

    c. "Your 5-year-old son may catch this as well."

    d. "Encourage her to drink plenty of orange juice."

14. The nurse is teaching a 14-year-old wrestler about the ringworm that he has contracted. Which of the following statements is the best advice to give this young man?

    a. "Be certain to take a shower after every practice and every meet."

    b. "You don't need to worry about giving this to your dog."

    c. "If you don't see any lesions on your teammates, they are safe."

    d. "When the lesions are gone, you can stop using the medicine."

15. Austin is a 7-yearold boy who is suffering from Stevens-Johnson syndrome. Which of the following interventions is most beneficial for him?

    a. Provide daily saline baths

    b. Use silver sulfadiazine cream as ordered

    c. Apply viscous lidocaine liberally to the oral cavity

    d. Recommend daily whirlpool treatments

16. Logan is a 4-year-old burn patient in the hospital who is due for his first dressing change in 1 hour. The nurse enters the room to discuss the procedure with the parents in the room. Which is the best statement for the nurse to make in regard to the forthcoming procedure?

    a. "You must leave the room for the procedure."

    b. "I will give him an oral pain medication just prior to his dressing change."

    c. "I will change his dressing as quickly as possible."

    d. "I will perform the dressing change here in his room."

17. Amber is a 2-year-old girl who is in the hospital for burns after pulling down a pot of hot water from the stove onto her chest. She was potty trained before the accident; however, she has been unable to hold her urine or stool since being admitted to the hospital. Which of the following would be the best interaction for the nurse to have with this child?

    a. "It is time to be a big girl and walk to the bathroom now."

    b. "It's okay for you to use a diaper while your burns get better."

    c. "We must use a diaper or your burns will hurt."

    d. "I know you used to use the potty before you were burned."

18. The nurse is caring for a 5-year-old boy with a major electrical injury. Which of the following statements would be most helpful when educating the parents about electrical injuries?

    a. "Myoglobinuria will cause your sons kidneys to fail."

    b. "You can see that the most damage is at the point of entry and point of exit."

    c. "Your child could have a serious arrhythmia as a result of the shock."

    d. "Your child will most likely not remember you were here today."

CHAPTER 26

The Child with Altered Endocrine Status

Learning Objectives

- Describe the functions of the endocrine system.
- Describe the symptoms associated with disorders of each endocrine gland.
- Identify diagnostic tests used to assess the disorders associated with each endocrine gland.
- Describe the interdisciplinary interventions unique to selected endocrine disorders, including the role of the nurse in managing the child's care.
- Describe the educational plan for a child with a newly diagnosed endocrine disorder that encompasses both acute healthcare needs and long-term home management needs.

SECTION I: ASSESSING YOUR UNDERSTANDING

Activity A *Match the description in column A with the appropriate answer in column B.*

Column A

___ 1. Polyphagia

___ 2. Menarche

___ 3. Thelarche

___ 4. Hyperfunction

___ 5. Adrenarche

Column B

a. Excessive hormone secretion

b. Excessive hunger

c. Growth of sexual hair

d. Breast development

e. Start of menstruation

Activity B *Match the altered endocrine function in column A with the correct definition in column B.*

Column A

___ 1. Pituitary gland

___ 2. Diabetes insipidus

___ 3. Syndrome of inappropriate antidiuretic hormone

___ 4. Hypopituitarism

___ 5. Precocious puberty

Column B

a. Disorder of the posterior pituitary that results from deficient secretion of ADH

b. Failure of the pituitary to produce sufficient growth hormone

c. Development of sexual characteristics before the usual age of puberty

d. Controls the release of at least seven different hormones

e. Secretion results from hypersecretion of ADH

Activity C *Place the following steps of negative feedback in their proper sequence.*

a. The target gland produces a hormone that inhibits the release of tropic hormone.

b. The tropic hormone affects another endocrine gland (target organ).

c. One endocrine gland produces a hormone (tropic hormone).

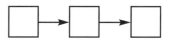

Activity D *Fill in the blanks.*

1. _____ is the lack of all anterior pituitary function.

2. Bottle-fed infants display symptoms of _____ _____ before breast-fed infants as a result of the hormones in breast milk.

3. _____ is rare in children, but can be fatal.

4. Parathyroid hormone hypersecretion by one or more of the parathyroid glands is called _____.

5. A child with _____ usually presents with the classic symptoms of polyuria and polydipsia.

SECTION II: APPLYING YOUR KNOWLEDGE

Activity E *Briefly answer the following.*

1. Discuss the possible pathophysiologic associations for type 2 diabetes.

   _____
   _____
   _____

2. What are the possible relations between environmental triggers and Addison's disease?

   _____
   _____
   _____

3. Discuss the effects of prolonged adrenal hyperplasia.

   _____
   _____
   _____

Activity F *Consider the scenario and answer the questions.*

Jesse is a 15-year-old boy who is being seen in the office today for a follow-up visit after being recently diagnosed with diabetes. He was brought to the hospital in the first place because he thought that he had strep throat.

1. He asks you at his visit today why "all of the sudden" did he get this. What is your response?

   _____
   _____

2. Jesse is confused regarding what is happening to his body and he wants to know why he cannot get the sugar that he needs from what he is eating. What would you tell him?

   _____
   _____

3. Jesse would like to know some of the long-term complications of type 1 diabetes? What would you tell him?

   _____
   _____

SECTION III: PRACTICING FOR NCLEX

Activity G *Choose the best answer.*

1. A nurse provides medication instructions to the parents, and a patient who is taking Synthroid. The nurse instructs the patient to notify the physician if which of the following occur?
   a. Cold intolerance
   b. Tremors
   c. Excessively dry skin
   d. Fatigue

2. When assessing regulatory function in a client, the action of which hormone produced by the pituitary gland needs to be evaluated by the nurse?
   a. Growth hormone
   b. Insulin
   c. Vasopressin
   d. Cortisol

3. The nurse recognizes that lowered blood glucose stimulates the release of which hormone from the pancreas?
   a. Glucocorticoid
   b. Cortisol
   c. Glucagon
   d. Glycogen

4. When assessing parathyroid function, the nurse monitors which of the following laboratory values?
   a. Magnesium
   b. Sodium
   c. Potassium
   d. Calcium

5. The nurse is assessing a 17-year-old girl who is in the office because she has not started menstruating. Which of the following endocrine glands is most often affected by age-related changes?
   a. Parathyroid
   b. Adrenal glands
   c. Thyroid
   d. Anterior pituitary

6. A 10-year-old is being seen in the office and has hyperthyroidism. The nurse knows that the most common cause of hyperthyroidism is which of the following?
   a. Addison's disease
   b. Cushing's disease
   c. Graves' disease
   d. Plummer's disease

7. The nurse is examining a child with hypoparathyroidism. The nurse is assessing for the presence of which sign?
   a. Paricalcitol
   b. Polyphagia
   c. Chvostek
   d. Troussaner's

8. Kenny, a 20-year-old, is being seen today for complaints of being tired, thirsty, and going to the bathroom frequently. Which of the following would indicate a need for diabetes testing?
   a. "My mother had gestational diabetes when she was pregnant with me."
   b. "My family is not as active as I am."
   c. "I exercise three to four times a week."
   d. "I do not take medications for blood pressure or cholesterol."

9. Becky is being seen today for issues associated with Addison's disease. The nurse knows that in an adolescent, this is associated with what other disease process?
   a. Cushing's disease
   b. Type 1 diabetes
   c. Graves' disease
   d. Type 2 diabetes

10. Ben is a 14-year-old who is being seen today for his asthma and rapid increase in weight. The nurse suspects that they are going to test for which of the following?
    a. Graves' disease
    b. Rainer's disease
    c. Cushing's syndrome
    d. Addison's disease

The Child with Inborn Errors of Metabolism

Learning Objectives

- Differentiate between inborn errors of metabolism that manifest at birth or in the immediate neonatal period (i.e., maple syrup disease) and those with later childhood onset (i.e., Wilson's disease).
- Describe key assessment factors that can assist in early identification of metabolic disorders in children.
- Describe interventions performed by the health-care team that are related to early identification of selected inborn errors of metabolism.
- State the dietary management specific to each metabolic disorder that can prevent disease symptoms or decrease their severity.
- Identify nursing interventions that assist the family and community to provide optimal care to the child with an inborn error of metabolism.

SECTION I: ASSESSING YOUR UNDERSTANDING

Activity A *Fill in the blanks.*

1. The body builds and maintains itself by _____ the food and fluid it ingests.

2. _____ _____ programs provide early diagnosis for many of the more common metabolic disorders.

3. _____ _____ is the primary goal in diagnostic evaluation for inborn errors of metabolism.

4. Neonatal screening tests for _____ and galactosemia are commonly mandated by state law.

5. The pattern of heredity for many of the metabolic conditions is _____, with neither parent presenting with clinically signs or symptoms.

Activity B *Match the terms related to metabolic disorders listed in column A with their definitions listed in column B.*

Column A

____ 1. Carrier testing

____ 2. Opisthotonos

____ 3. Ceruloplasmin

____ 4. Rachitic

____ 5. Poikilothermia

____ 6. Kayser-Fleischer rings

Column B

a. Glycoprotein, to which most of the copper in the blood is attached

b. Extreme spasmic extension of the body resulting in arching of the back at a severe angle

c. Inability to maintain a consistent core body temperature

d. Individuals affected by rickets

e. Heterozygote screening

f. Corneal copper deposits around the iris

Activity C *Briefly answer the following.*

1. Explain why identifying the cause and symptoms of metabolic disturbances accurately and quickly is essential.

   _____

   _____

   _____

2. List the abnormalities commonly revealed in a physical examination focused on evaluating neurodevelopmental functions.

   _____

   _____

   _____

3. Give three examples of specific criteria that must be met before a metabolic disorder is included in a neonatal screening program.

   _____

   _____

   _____

4. List four laboratory studies that are used to analyze blood, plasma, urine, or cerebrospinal fluid to detect metabolic disorders.

   _____

   _____

   _____

5. Give three situations in which a healthcare team should consider and suspect a metabolic disorder.

   _____

   _____

   _____

6. Describe three treatment interventions for a metabolic disorder.

   _____

   _____

   _____

Activity D *Match the definitions in column A with the disorders listed in column B.*

Column A

_____ 1. Its hallmark is an extreme copper deficiency

_____ 2. Hereditary, X-linked dominant, renal phosphate wasting disorder

_____ 3. Classic and most severe form of mucopolysaccharidosis type I

_____ 4. Autosomal recessive disorder of copper metabolism characterized by cirrhosis of the liver and degenerative changes in the brain

_____ 5. Rare inherited metabolic disorder in which the body is unable to metabolize galactose

Column B

a. Galactosemia

b. Menkes

c. Hurler's

d. Rickets

e. Wilson's

SECTION II: APPLYING YOUR KNOWLEDGE

Activity E *Consider the scenario and answer the questions.*

The hospital nurse brings Joshua, a 2-day-old infant, to his mother, Rebecca, for breast-feeding. When the father greets the nurse at the door, the nurse recognizes the distinctive dress and dialect of the local Mennonite group living in the community. Rebecca appears anxious about breast-feeding and tells the nurse that Joshua has been "fussy" and "spitting up milk." She also states that Joshua "smells different" today than he did yesterday and she asks the nurse if she was doing something wrong with breast-feeding him. The nurse checks the infant's chart and notices that a Guthrie test has been performed, but the results are not back yet.

1. Based on this information, which metabolic disorder would the nurse suspect? What further testing should be performed to diagnose this disorder?

   _____

   _____

2. What interdisciplinary interventions should be instituted if Joshua is diagnosed with the suspected metabolic disorder?

_____

_____

3. What family-centered nursing interventions could the nurse institute to support the family through this crisis?

_____

_____

SECTION III: PRACTICING FOR NCLEX

Activity F *Choose the best answer.*

1. The culturally competent nurse screens for certain metabolic disorders that are known to be more prevalent in specific ethnic geographic groups. For example, a high prevalence of Tay-Sachs disease occurs more frequently among individuals of what descent?
   a. Jews of Yemenite origin
   b. French Canadians
   c. Ashkenazi Jewish individuals
   d. Mennonite and Amish sects

2. The neonatal nurse changing the diaper of a neonate notices a musty, mousy smell. The nurse knows that this smell may be indicative of which of the following?
   a. Hypermethioninemia
   b. Phenylketonuria
   c. Multiple carboxylase deficiency
   d. Hawkinsinuria

3. The parents of an infant diagnosed with hemochromatosis asks the nurse what caused this condition in their baby. What is the nurse's best response?
   a. "Hemochromatosis is an accumulation of iron that can cause extensive tissue damage if not treated."
   b. "Hemochromatosis is caused by a systemic zinc deficiency that will cause progressive deterioration if not treated."

   c. "Hemochromatosis occurs as a result of intestinal malabsorption of magnesium and can be well controlled with management is maintained."
   d. "Hemochromatosis is caused by a deficit of alpha-galactosidase and, in most cases, renal treatment can reverse the symptoms."

4. Based on laboratory findings of elevated acid phosphatase and lipid-laden cells found in the bone marrow, a doctor diagnoses a patient with Gaucher's disease. The nurse is aware that this condition is caused by which of the following?
   a. Deficient sphingomyelinase
   b. Deficient hexosaminidase A
   c. Deficient iduronate sulfatase
   d. Deficient beta-glucosidase

5. A nurse studying the laboratory results of a patient documents elevations in BUN creatinine. The nurse is aware that these elevations are indicative of which of the following?
   a. Renal involvement
   b. Hepatic involvement
   c. Cardiac involvement
   d. Neurologic involvement

6. A pediatric nurse explains to the parents of an infant with mitochondrial disease that alterations have occurred in which type of tissue?
   a. Skin
   b. Muscle
   c. Liver
   d. Cardiac

7. A nurse planning a diet for a patient with Wilson's disease knows that treatment for Wilson's disease commonly involves following a low-copper diet. Which one of the following foods is low in copper?
   a. Salmon
   b. Tofu
   c. White-meat chicken
   d. Mushrooms

8. The pediatric nurse caring for children with metabolic disorders knows that which of the following inborn error of metabolism occurs during the neonatal period?

   a. Hurler's syndrome

   b. Hunter's syndrome

   c. Wilson's disease

   d. Galactosemia

9. The parents of 11-year-old Jonnie, diagnosed with phenylketonuria (PKU), tell the nurse that Jonnie has told them that she hates "being different from the other kids and being teased about eating weird foods." What is an appropriate intervention to teach the parents regarding Jonnie's diet compliance?

   a. Sit down with Jonnie and explain her condition and need for the diet

   b. Let the parents determine when the medical food will be taken

   c. Ask the teacher to answer questions from other students about Jonnie's diet

   d. Provide genetic counseling and information regarding the risks of a PKU pregnancy

10. The neonatal nurse reviews the guidelines for completing neonatal screening established by her hospital. Which of the following is an appropriate neonatal screening guideline?

    a. Newborn screening should be completed prior to 10 days of life

    b. Screening of premature infants should be competed by the seventh day of life

    c. Screening should be completed after transfusion or dialysis

    d. Screening should be completed preferably between 24 and 72 hours of age

Activity G *Choose all answers that apply.*

1. The pediatric nurse caring for infants in a family-centered healthcare facility screens patients for the signs of the existence of a metabolic disorder. These signs include which of the following?

   a. Rejection of carbohydrates

   b. Failure to thrive

   c. Delayed development

   d. History of poor feeding

   e. History of infections

   f. Vision or hearing loss

2. A neonate is diagnosed with tyrosinemia type I. The nurse knows that which of the following are clinical manifestations of this disorder?

   a. Mental retardation

   b. Liver cirrhosis

   c. Lethargy

   d. Bloody stools

   e. Jaundice

   f. Acidosis

Activity H *Fill in the blanks.*

1. The nurse caring for patients with metabolic disorders knows that the goal of dietary restriction, the primary treatment modality for inborn errors of metabolism, is to control the substrate accumulation by reducing or eliminating carbohydrates, proteins, or both. Special diet restrictions and synthetic _____ _____ are the two most successful methods of controlling the enzyme deficiencies.

2. The nurse researcher knows that in _____ _____, normal genetic information is introduced into defective cells to compensate for genetic defects and to correct disease phenotypes.

3. The nurse explains to parents of an infant with a metabolic disorder that _____ is the most frequently occurring aminoaciduria.

The Child with Altered Sensory Status

Learning Objectives

- Identify deviations from normal developmental patterns that indicate a visual, hearing, or communication disorder.
- Describe assessment techniques commonly used to identify vision, hearing, and communication disorders in infants and children.
- Identify the nursing interventions necessary to prepare children and their families for tests of sensory function.
- Describe the etiology of common vision, hearing, and communication disorders of infants and children.
- Discuss the pathophysiology related to common disorders of vision, hearing, and communication in infancy and childhood.
- Identify the roles of the interdisciplinary team members in identifying and managing sensory disorders in children.
- Develop a plan of care for an infant or child with an alteration in vision, hearing, or communication.
- Summarize parent and child education to prevent injuries and illness resulting in alterations in sensory function.

SECTION I: ASSESSING YOUR UNDERSTANDING

Activity A *Match the alteration in vision in column A with the proper phrase or term in column B.*

Column A

_____ **1.** Refractive errors

_____ **2.** Myopia

_____ **3.** Hyperopia

_____ **4.** Astigmatism

_____ **5.** Strabismus

_____ **6.** Amblyopia

Column B

a. Poor vision for distant objects

b. Accommodation and convergence

c. Esotropia and exotropia

d. Obstructions to ?vision

e. Farsightedness

f. Irregular curvature of cornea

Activity B *Match the alteration in hearing in column A with phrase or term in column B.*

Column A

_____ **1.** Otitis media

_____ **2.** Otitis externa

_____ **3.** Conductive hearing impairment

_____ **4.** Central hearing impairment

_____ **5.** Sensorineural hearing impairment

Column B

a. Distorted and lost sounds

b. Outer or middle ear

c. Upper respiratory infection

d. Brain damage

e. Alcohol and vinegar drops

Activity C *Place the following developmental stages for vision in the proper order.*

a. Binocular vision is achieved.
b. Eye can change shape to focus.
c. Fix vision on an object.
d. Follow a moving object.

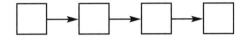

Activity D *Fill in the blanks.*

1. The results of Rinne's and Weber tests may not be _____ when assessing children younger than 8 years of age.

2. The _____ of sound is measured in decibels.

3. The auditory brain stem response test compensates for a child's inability to _____ with hearing test procedure.

4. An infant who had cataracts removed should be examined for eye pain and _____ if he is irritable for no apparent reason or is rubbing his eyes.

5. Ophthalmia neonatorum, also called neonatal _____, may be caused by bacterial or viral infection or chemicals.

6. Audiometry measures two characteristics of sound: _____ and _____.

7. Hearing and listening form the foundation for _____.

8. _____ is a common symptom in voice disorders.

SECTION II: APPLYING YOUR KNOWLEDGE

Activity E *Briefly answer the following.*

1. What are the four ways in which nurses facilitate screening and prevention of vision, hearing, and communication disorders?

_____

_____

_____

2. Describe the difference between a speech disorder and a language disorder.

_____

_____

_____

3. Describe the difference between conductive and sensorineural hearing loss, including the roles that intensity and pitch play, and how hearing aids and cochlear implants are used.

_____

_____

_____

4. Discuss the issues that a child with multiple deficits faces and how to deal with such issues.

_____

_____

_____

Activity F *Consider the scenario and answer the questions.*

John, who is 5 years old, has just started kindergarten. His teacher notes that he has difficulty recognizing objects that are placed on the chalkboard in the front of the classroom. He often squints or closes his left eye when he is trying to read or look at books. She sends a letter home to John's mother and refers him to the school nurse. As the school nurse evaluating John, answer the following questions.

1. What would be the key points of your assessment of John?

_____

_____

2. You note on your assessment that John's left eye is not able to track the pencil and hold the position. He keeps trying to cover his left eye when reading the visual acuity chart. You refer him to an ophthalmologist who diagnoses him with amblyopia. John will be undergoing occlusion therapy and will wear an eye patch to school every day. As the school nurse, what responsibilities would you have when caring for John?

_____

_____

3. John's mother is concerned how his diagnosis and treatment will affect his vision in the future. What would you tell her?

_____

_____

SECTION III: PRACTICING FOR NCLEX

Activity G *Choose the best answer.*

1. The nurse is taking a health history for a 9-year-old child with red, runny eyes. Which of the following findings would suggest that this is infectious conjunctivitis?
   a. A playmate had pink eye
   b. Known allergy to dust mites
   c. Recent cerumen impaction
   d. Family history of conjunctivitis

2. The nurse is assessing an infant with ophthalmia neonatorum. Which of the following findings indicate the need to alert the doctor?
   a. Inflammation of the eyelids
   b. Poor feeding and irritability
   c. Purulent discharge from the eyes
   d. Edema of the eyelids

3. The nurse is performing a physical assessment for a 1-week-old infant. Which of the following findings suggests the possibility of glaucoma?
   a. White, opaque appearance of the lens
   b. Absence of the red reflex
   c. The sclera appear blue
   d. Copious, purulent drainage

4. The nurse is caring for a 6-year-old child who has been diagnosed with myopia. Which of the following describes the pathophysiology of the child's eyes?
   a. Shorter than normal axial length
   b. Asymmetric cornea curvature
   c. Greatly divergent refractive errors
   d. Light rays focus in front of the retina

5. The nurse is performing a physical assessment for a 14-year-old girl with an ear ache. Which of the following signs and symptoms indicates acute otitis externa?
   a. The tympanic membrane reacts to a puff of air
   b. Symptoms of upper respiratory infection are present
   c. The ear canal is devoid of cerumen
   d. The area around the tragus is tender to the touch

6. The nurse is completing a health history of a 5-year-old boy with amblyopia. Which of the following is most likely to be a finding?
   a. Chemical conjunctivitis at birth
   b. A recent mild eye injury
   c. Mother was drug dependent
   d. Frequent upper respiratory infections

7. The nurse is teaching parents of a 4-year-old boy about otitis media. Which of the following statements represents correct teaching by the nurse?
   a. "Tobacco smoke exposure is not related to ear infections.
   b. "Children's eustachian tubes are long and narrow."
   c. "This is unusual for a child this age."
   d. "Ear infection frequently follows a head cold."

8. The nurse is providing home care instructions to the mother of a 6-year-old child with infectious conjunctivitis. Which of the following instructions will best help prevent the spread of infection within the family?
   a. "Use all the medication as directed."
   b. "The whole family should wash hands frequently."
   c. "This could have started with a head cold."
   d. "Place the ointment inside the lower eyelid."

9. During the physical assessment of a 14-year-old child who had a previous eye injury, the nurse becomes concerned that the child may have a cataract in the eye. Which of the following signs or symptoms supports the nurse's concern?

    a. Ptosis of the eyelids

    b. Complaints of eye itching

    c. Absence of the red reflex

    d. Edema of the eyelids

10. The nurse is educating the parents of a newborn with conjunctivitis. Which of the following comments will be part of the information provided?

    a. "This can be genetic or acquired."

    b. "It's an overgrowth of retinal blood vessels."

    c. "The liquid inside the eye can't drain."

    d. "This is often caused by silver nitrate."

The Child with Altered Mental Health

Learning Objectives

- Describe the mental status examination and the techniques used to assess alterations in children's mental health.
- Explain the purpose and the use of the interdisciplinary categories (from the *Diagnostic and Statistical Manual of Mental Disorders*) used to diagnose, communicate, and treat alterations in children and adolescents' mental health.
- Identify the criteria that indicate a need to refer children and adolescents to mental health professionals.
- Describe interventions used to treat altered mental health in children and adolescents.
- Describe the relation between cultural variables and alterations in mental health.
- Discuss the influence of growth and development in relation to altered mental health.
- Describe the behavioral, emotional, physical, and cognitive effects of abuse and neglect.

SECTION I: ASSESSING YOUR UNDERSTANDING

Activity A *Match the key term in column A with the correct definition in column B.*

Column A

____ 1. Hallucinations

____ 2. Affect

____ 3. Delusional thought

____ 4. Dissociation

____ 5. Mania

Column B

a. External expression of emotion attached to the ideas or representation of objects

b. Sensory impressions, such as sights, sounds, tastes, or smells, that have no basis in external stimulation

c. A phase of bipolar disorder characterized by expansiveness, elation, agitation, hyperexcitability, hyperactivity, and increase speed of thought or speech

d. False beliefs that are firmly maintained despite proof to the contrary

e. A defense mechanism in which a group of mental processes is segregated from the rest of a person's mental processes to avoid emotional distress

Activity B *Match the psychotropic medication classification in column A with an example of this medication in column B.*

Column A

____ 1. Stimulant

____ 2. Tricyclic antidepressant

Column B

a. Olanzapine (Zyprexa)

b. Buspirone

c. Lithium

____ **3.** Monoamine oxidase inhibitor antidepressant

____ **4.** Selective serotonin reuptake inhibitors antidepressant

____ **5.** Antimanic agents

____ **6.** Seizure medications

____ **7.** Antianxiety agents

____ **8.** Noradrenergic agents

____ **9.** Antipsychotic agents

____ **10.** Atypical antipsychotics

d. Ritalin

e. Fluoxetine (Prozac)

f. Tegretol

g. Amitriptyline (Elavil)

h. Thorazine

i. Imipramine

j. Clonidine

Activity C *Place the following steps in the cognitive behavior therapeutic process in the proper order.*

a. Help patients see the relations among their thoughts and beliefs, and their emotional responses.

b. Understand the patient's cognitive system.

c. Encourage patients to use problem solving to identify alternative solutions or ways of behaving.

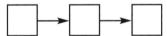

Activity D *Fill in the blanks.*

1. Risk for _____ is dramatically elevated in depressed youth.

2. A depressed or irritable mood that is less intense and more persistent than major depression is called _____.

3. Anxiety in children, regardless of age or gender, often manifests in _____ complaints such as headaches or stomachaches.

4. To confirm a diagnosis of separation anxiety disorder, the symptoms must have been present for at least _____ weeks.

5. Pictures of _____ are often shown to children who are in treatment because they refuse to go to school to indicate the amount of fear experienced and to evaluate progress.

6. Because of the potential for reactionary aggressive behavior in posttraumatic stress disorder, it is commonly confused with _____ disorder.

7. Levels of melatonin and _____ are strongly correlated with the incidence of seasonal affective disorder.

8. One out of _____ children and adolescents struggles with some form of emotional, behavioral, or mental illness.

9. _____ therapy is based on the assumptions that thoughts mediate behavior.

10. _____ is a mental illness that manifests itself by extreme changes in mood, activity, and behavior.

Activity E *Name each of the five axes of the DSM-IV diagnostic classifications.*

Axis I: _____, _____

Axis II: _____, _____

Axis III: _____

Axis IV: _____, _____

Axis V: _____

SECTION II: APPLYING YOUR KNOWLEDGE

Activity F *Briefly answer the questions.*

1. Is *conduct disorder* another term for *delinquency*? Explain.

_____

_____

2. Describe oppositional defiant disorder.

_____

_____

3. Describe a common way for youth to communicate about suicide. Cite an example.

_____

_____

4. Define substance abuse.

_____

_____

Activity G *Consider the scenario and answer the questions.*

Marisa is a 10-year-old who is being seen today because her parents have scheduled an appointment because of her recent acting out at home and in school. Her parents separated more than a year ago and have been dating other people who they have been introduced into Marisa's life.

1. What important information needs to be collected during the mental status examination?

_____

_____

2. Through all the examinations and assessments, it is determined that Marisa has always been more negative, hostile, and argumentative than other children her age. It is determined that Marisa had oppositional defiant disorder (ODD). Why is it important to assess Marisa for depression as well?

_____

_____

3. Marisa's parents ask about potential outcomes for children with ODD. What education should be given?

_____

_____

SECTION III: PRACTICING FOR THE NCLEX

Activity H *Choose the best answer.*

1. A 17-year-old boy has recently been diagnosed with schizophrenia and is being discharged from a residential treatment facility. His parents express their remorse to the nurse over what they might have done wrong to contribute to his illness. How should the nurse respond?
   a. Advise the parents that the onset of schizophrenia is insidious
   b. Tell them that an accurate diagnosis can take several years
   c. Tell them that they need to be strong for their son
   d. Assuage the parents' guilt and refer them to a support group

2. A school nurse sees a 13-year-old female student in her office for a sore throat. The nurse notices that the child has eroded dental enamel and reddened and inflamed gums. She does not have a fever. This alerts the nurse to the possibility of bulimia. What should the nurse say next?
   a. "Will you please step on the scale? I need to make a note of your weight."
   b. "Do you know what bulimia is?"
   c. "Have you noticed that the enamel on your teeth is eroding?
   d. "How long has your throat been bothering you?"

3. A 9-year-old boy is experiencing a panic attack on the playground. The playground supervisor brings the boy to the school nurse's office. What should the nurse do first?
   a. Encourage him to breathe deeply and visualize a comforting object or thought
   b. Calmly call the children's parents and request their assistance
   c. Quietly ask the playground supervisor what precipitated the attack
   d. Tell the child that everything is going to be okay

4. An 8-year-old girl has refused to board the school bus several times during the past 6 weeks. Recently, she refused to disembark from the bus when it arrived at the school and had to be coaxed off by school staff. The girl's parents are recently divorced. The mother has called the school nurse because she believes that everyone is treating her daughter too harshly. What should the school nurse say to the mother?

   a. "Your daughter might have separation anxiety."

   b. "Let's try to work together to help your daughter."

   c. "What concerns you about your daughter's treatment at school?"

   d. "What do you think is going on with your daughter?"

5. A 7-year-old girl is being treated for an anxiety disorder. The nurse is working with the girl to provide appropriate stress reduction techniques. Which of the following would be the best way to introduce the most appropriate nursing intervention to the girl?

   a. "Let's think of your favorite place to visit and take a trip there in our minds."

   b. "Tell me about your favorite game you play in physical education class."

   c. "Let's write some positive affirmations on these sticky notes for you to take home."

   d. "Tell me what you think you can do better to avoid stress."

6. A 10-year-old boy is receiving medication for an anxiety disorder. His parents have set up a meeting with the Advanced Practice Psychiatric Nurse Practitioner to seek a second opinion, because they do not think he is getting better. Which of the following statements would be most helpful to educate the parents about this disorder?

   a. "It is important to realize that not everyone responds to medications."

   b. "It is important understand as much as possible about the disorder."

   c. "It is important for you comfortable with the treatment plan and goals."

   d. "It is important for your son to receive therapy as well as medication."

7. The nurse is caring for an 11-year-old girl hospitalized for injuries sustained in a motor vehicle accident. The girl's mother died as a result of her injuries. What action would be most appropriate in this situation?

   a. Inform the girl that her mother passed away

   b. Implement crisis intervention and family support measures

   c. Contact the girl's teachers

   d. Schedule a session with a cognitive behavioral therapist

8. The nurse is caring for a 13-year-old girl with anorexia nervosa. Which of the following questions would be most helpful to elicit the child's perception of her body image?

   a. "Do you think you look healthy at this weight?"

   b. "Did you know that you could suffer permanent damage?"

   c. "What do you see when you look in the mirror?"

   d. "Do you like what you see when you look in the mirror?"

9. The parents of a 4-year-old enlisted the assistance of the nurse to help the child with a sleep disorder. The child refused to go to bed at night in her own bed. The child had no mental alterations. It has been a week since the parents initiated the suggested interventions and they are frustrated that the problem is not solved. What would be the most appropriate response to their concerns?

   a. Advise the parents to keep a night light on

   b. Remind the parents to leave the child's bedroom door open

   c. Remind the parents to keep their expectations reasonable

   d. Advise the parents to avoid excessive anger and abusive discipline

10. The nurse is caring for a 16-year-old boy with a conduct disorder. He is hospitalized after intentionally cutting himself with a piece of broken glass. When the nurse collects his pencil after a group therapy session, the boy becomes upset and uses abusive language. How should the nurse respond?

   a. "I don't make the rules here; I just enforce them."

   b. "I understand your frustration, but the unit rule is to collect all pencils."

   c. "I am concerned that you might hurt yourself."

   d. "I will let you keep the pencil for 15 more minutes."

The Child with a Developmental or Learning Disorder

Learning Objectives

- Discuss adaptive functional and educational responses of children with a developmental disorder.
- Explain the importance of early identification and intervention with children who have a developmental disorder.
- Discuss strategies to help parents navigate the healthcare system and advocate for their child to ensure that their child receives needed healthcare.
- Identify strategies for including a child with a developmental disorder in typical environments in the community.
- Support families in their efforts to identify and use community resources that best meet the individual child's and family's needs.

SECTION I: ASSESSING YOUR UNDERSTANDING

Activity A *Match the test name in column A with the proper phrase in column B.*

Column A

___ 1. Bayley-III

___ 2. Stanford-Binet

___ 3. Vineland Adaptive Behavior Scales

Column B

a. Identify strengths and weaknesses

b. Measures personal and social skills

___ 4. Wechsler Preschool/Primary Scale of Intelligence

___ 5. Wechsler Intelligence Scale for Children

c. Has 15 subtests of ?various abilities

d. Has four index scores for IQ

e. Cognitive, language, and motor scales

Activity B *Match the diagnostic modality in column A with the correct phrase in column B.*

Column A

___ 1. Computed tomography

___ 2. Fluorescent in situ hybridization

___ 3. Heavy metal assay

___ 4. Magnetic resonance imaging

___ 5. Metabolic screening

Column B

a. Venous sample preferred

b. Three-dimensional view of structures

c. Detects inborn errors

d. Information about tissue chemistry

e. Genetic abnormalities

Activity C *Fill in the blanks.*

1. A successful plan of care focuses on the _____ and resilience of the child's family.

2. Learning disorders do not predict _____ or learning capabilities.

114

3. Assessment of a child with mental retardation should focus on _____ ability.

4. A key role for the nurse is as an _____ for the child to obtain services and care.

5. Children with autism show little _____ for others and do not respond to affection.

6. Lack of _____ and _____ may permanently alter brain development.

7. The _____ is always critical for a complete assessment.

8. Failure to achieve developmental _____ may indicate a developmental disorder.

9. Tests of cognitive and _____ functioning help to diagnose developmental disorders.

10. Children with learning disorders are susceptible to _____ and _____.

SECTION II: APPLYING YOUR KNOWLEDGE

Activity D *Briefly answer the following.*

1. What are the disorders that belong in the category of autism?

   _____

   _____

   _____

2. Name six problem areas experienced by children with learning disorders.

   _____

   _____

   _____

3. How does the ability to think abstractly affect the mentally retarded child?

   _____

   _____

   _____

4. List some of the possible causes of developmental disorders.

   _____

   _____

   _____

5. Why is the term *cognitive functioning* more appropriate than *intelligence* when testing children?

   _____

   _____

   _____

Activity E *Consider the scenario and answer the questions.*

Kendall, age 3 years, was diagnosed with autism 3 months earlier. His family recently moved to Florida from North Carolina and his parents are still struggling with dealing with the diagnosis. This is their first visit to Kendall's new clinic, and his parents report that, during the past week, Kendall has become increasingly frustrated and has started throwing temper tantrums and banging his head on the wall. Kendall's mother is very worried and states, "I just don't know what to do. Kendall was doing so well before we moved and now he seems to have gone backward."

1. What would you say to Kendall's mother regarding her concerns?

   _____

   _____

2. What interdisciplinary strategies would be appropriate to introduce at this time?

   _____

   _____

3. Because they are new to the area, what resources could you provide for this family?

   _____

   _____

SECTION III: PRACTICING FOR NCLEX

Activity F *Choose the best answer.*

1. The nurse is observing a 4-year-old boy suspected of having autistic disorder. Which of the following signs and symptoms are consistent with Asperger's syndrome?

   a. Has below-average intellectual function

   b. Shows signs of losing attained skills

   c. Performs repetitive activity with toys

   d. Possesses excellent language development

2. The nurse is educating the parents of a 9-year-old girl about her learning disorder. Which of the following facts would be included in the discussion?

 a. Learning disorders indicate lower intelligence

 b. Learning disorders are, in fact, learning deficits

 c. The disorder requires comprehensive special education

 d. The child may have unusual talent in another area

3. The nurse is caring for a 5-year-old girl who may have a developmental disorder. Which of the following would suggest that she does?

 a. The child repeatedly slaps herself on the head

 b. The child must be supervised when brushing her teeth

 c. The child knows what a dog and a cat sound like

 d. The child has trouble with "r," "l," and "y" sounds

4. The nurse is preparing a plan to educate the parents of a 9-year-old boy with a learning disorder. Which of the following will be part of this plan?

 a. Encourage the parents to give the child personal space

 b. Tell the parents to check on the child regularly

 c. Teach the parents about the child's specific difficulty

 d. Have the parents learn the child's facial expressions

5. The nurse is performing a physical assessment of a 4-year-old girl with Down syndrome. Which of the following signs and symptoms is typical of the disorder?

 a. Large ears

 b. Long face

 c. Upward slanted palpebral fissures

 d. Flat, recessed forehead

6. The nurse is caring for a 9-year-old boy with a developmental disorder. Which of the following is an example of impaired adaptive functioning?

 a. The child cannot correctly copy a phone number

 b. The child uses a system of sign language and grunts

 c. The child's vision is fine but he reads very poorly

 d. The child cannot correctly copy a sentence

7. The nurse is teaching self-care skills to an 11-year-old mentally retarded child. Which of the following techniques are unique to this teaching situation?

 a. Being consistent with expectations

 b. Avoiding abstract descriptions

 c. Individualizing the teaching methods

 d. Being patient and rewarding successes

8. The nurse is caring for a 6-year-old girl with mental retardation who is scheduled for a chromosomal analysis. Which of the following comments would help prepare her and her mother for the procedure?

 a. "We need to discuss her diet before the test."

 b. "We'll give you a pill that makes you sleepy."

 c. "You're going to lay down and listen to music."

 d. "We'll numb her arm before we try to draw blood."

9. The nurse has completed the health history and physical assessment of a 6-year-old boy and further diagnostic tests are required. Which of the following activities will the nurse do next?

 a. Perform the Wechsler Intelligence Scales test

 b. Provide genetic counseling

 c. Help the parents interpret the test results

 d. Administer the Stanford-Binet test

10. The nurse is preparing an education plan to help the family learn about their child's developmental disorder and its treatment. Which of the following interventions will be part of the plan?

 a. Providing education to build social skills

 b. Conducting developmental assessments of the child

 c. Teaching how to plan schedules and routines

 d. Linking the family to support groups

CHAPTER 31

Pediatric Emergencies

Learning Objectives

- Describe the four components of pediatric emergency triage.
- Describe the nursing interventions required for the infant or child in cardiopulmonary arrest.
- Discuss common causes, signs, and symptoms of shock in children.
- Prioritize the sequence of assessing the multiple-trauma patient.
- Identify common signs of and management for hypoxia in a child in respiratory distress.
- Explain the physiologic effects of fever in a child.
- Describe the nursing interventions for the child who has been bitten or stung.
- Discuss management of anaphylaxis.
- Describe the initial nursing intervention for a child with epistaxis.
- Discuss the nursing interventions for the child with an environmental injury: hypothermia, hyperthermia, or near drowning.
- Identify the initial treatment for the child who has ingested an unknown poison.
- Discuss nursing interventions for a family whose child has died of sudden infant death syndrome (SIDS).
- Discuss considerations for interfacility transfer.

SECTION I: ASSESSING YOUR UNDERSTANDING

Activity A *Match the term in column A with the correct description in column B.*

Column A

_____ 1. Hypovolemic

_____ 2. Cardiogenic

_____ 3. Distributive

_____ 4. Obstructive

Column B

a. Impaired pumping ability

b. Inadequate cardiac output

c. Loss of fluid and electrolytes

d. Sepsis

Activity B *Fill in the blanks.*

1. The cause of SIDS is _____.

2. Certain compounds are used to bind with metallic poisons in a process called _____ therapy.

3. More people die of _____ _____ than burn injuries within the first 24 hours.

4. _____ is the inherited tendency to form immunoglobulin E antibodies.

Activity C *Briefly answer the following.*

1. List the steps for primary and secondary assessment.

   _____

   _____

   _____

2. Explain the significance of "raccoon eyes" and the possible risks to the child.

   _____

   _____

   _____

3. In an emergency trauma situation, identify what must be completed before administering pain medication.

_____

_____

_____

SECTION II: APPLYING YOUR KNOWLEDGE

Activity D *Consider the following scenario and answer the questions.*

Caroline Tierney brings her 4-year-old daughter, Crystal, to the emergency department. Caroline states, "She was fine just a couple of hours ago. Then she got a fever and started having trouble breathing. I can't get her to eat or drink anything." Assessment reveals the following: temperature, 104.4 °F (40.2 °C); tripod positioning; and a cough with stridor. Epiglottitis is suspected.

1. How do Crystal's signs and symptoms differ from those that would be associated with croup?

_____

_____

2. What interventions would the nurse expect to implement for Crystal?

_____

_____

SECTION III: PRACTICING FOR NCLEX

Activity E *Choose the best answer.*

1. The nurse is caring for a 2-year-old child who has swallowed an unknown number of acetaminophen tablets earlier in the day. Which action would be performed first?
   a. Administering N-acetylcysteine
   b. Initiating chelation therapy
   c. Starting IV fluid replacement
   d. Performing a gastric lavage

2. A 9-month-old child with trauma has arrived in the emergency department. Which of the following actions will the nurse take after assessing the ABC status?
   a. Assessing metabolic demands
   b. Maintaining proper core temperature
   c. Checking level of consciousness
   d. Assessing vital signs

3. The nurse is caring for a 1-year-old girl with a 102 °F temperature and toxic appearance. Which of the following would be the primary intervention?
   a. Administering prescribed IV antibiotics promptly
   b. Performing a complete septic workup
   c. Obtaining a specimen for a complete blood count
   d. Replacing any fluid volume deficits

4. Parents have brought their 6-year-old boy to urgent care because they were unable to stop his nose from bleeding. The nurse cannot stop the bleeding by applying pressure. Which of the following would the nurse expect to assist with next?
   a. Applying a lidocaine-soaked plug
   b. Positioning the child with his head tilted back
   c. Applying petroleum jelly inside the nares
   d. Having the site cauterized with silver nitrate

5. A 12-year-old boy has broken his leg and is showing signs and symptoms of shock. Which of the following actions should the nurse take after providing 100% oxygen by mask?
   a. Check circulation in the toes of the affected leg
   b. Establish intravenous access
   c. Provide oral analgesics as ordered
   d. Position the boy on his back with his head elevated

6. The nurse had been caring for a 6-month-old baby who died of SIDS or child abuse. Which of the following signs supports abuse as the cause of death?
   a. The infant's face appears bruised
   b. Parents' histories are inconsistent
   c. There are signs of trauma on the body
   d. The baby's occiput is flattened

Answers

CHAPTER 1

SECTION I: ASSESSING YOUR UNDERSTANDING

Activity A FILL IN THE BLANKS.

1. Family-centered care
2. Family
3. Reproductive
4. Affective
5. Medical home
6. Crisis
7. Nuclear

Activity B MATCH THE FAMILY THEORY IN COLUMN A WITH ITS BASIC TENET LISTED IN COLUMN B.

1. c   2. a   3. e   4. b   5. d

Activity C BRIEFLY ANSWER THE FOLLOWING.

1. Sample definitions of family include
   - Family is whomever the person says it is (Bozett, 1987)
   - A group of individuals who are bound by strong emotional ties, a sense of belonging, and a passion for being involved in one another's lives (Wright, Watson & Bell, 1996)
   - A group of two or more persons related by blood, marriage, or adoption who are residing together (U.S. Census Bureau, 2004)
2. The developmental issues that may occur when deciding to divorce include accepting one's own part in the failure of the marriage and accepting the inability to resolve marital tensions sufficiently to continue.
3. Sample definitions of family-centered care include
   - The identification of problems and needs of a family and the provision of appropriate service for every family member (Yauger, 1972)
   - A philosophy, a way of approaching a family, rather than a set of procedures (Atkinson, 1976)
   - Viewing the family not as a collection of individuals, but as a discrete entity, as the fundamental

unit of medical care delivery (Schwenck & Hughes, 1983)

4. Issues related to international adoptions include
   - Child comes from "high-risk" background
   - Child lived in an institution prior to adoption
   - Child lacked nutritional food, clothing, and healthcare
   - Child presents with developmental delays
5. Strategies to support children and their adoptive families include
   - Preadoptive consultations with an international adoption specialist, who can help ascertain whether the referred child is one the family feels adequate to parent
   - A complete physical, developmental, and emotional evaluation to determine areas of concern
   - A screening of the child for infectious diseases acquired in the country of origin (e.g., tuberculosis, hepatitis B, HIV, hepatitis C, syphilis, and gastrointestinal pathogens) and specific diseases not previously screened (e.g., phenylketonuria and sickle cell anemia); previous screenings should not be considered reliable
   - A review of immunization records; if documentation is lacking, the child should be considered unimmunized and receive the full series of immunizations
6. Sample nursing interventions to enhance family-centered care include
   - Changing visiting policies to promote the presence of family at the bedside
   - Developing activities to support the family as they make the transition from one unit to another
   - Making sure there is an adequate number of sleeping cots for parents

Activity D MATCH THE DEFINITIONS IN COLUMN A WITH THE TERMS LISTED IN COLUMN B.

1. c   2. a   3. b   4. e   5. f
6. d

SECTION II: APPLYING YOUR KNOWLEDGE

Activity E **CONSIDER THIS SCENARIO AND ANSWER THE QUESTIONS.**

1. According the following definitions, Chad is a member of Melinda's family:

   ■ A family is two or more persons who are related in any way—biologically, legally, or emotionally. Patients and families define their families (Institute for Family Centered Care, 2007).

   ■ A family is a primary social group in any society, typically consisting of a man and a woman, or any two individuals who wish to share their lives together in a long-term commitment to one another, bring up offspring, and usually reside in the same dwelling (Maskanian, 2007).

   ■ A family is whomever the patient says it is (Bozett, 1987).

2. The nurse should view Chad and Melinda as members of a family that is a discrete entity and is the fundamental unit of medical care delivery. Services should be designed in response to the needs of Chad and his family, with the child, family, and service providers in an interactive system. The nurse should facilitate collaboration at all levels of hospital, home, and community care, and should exchange complete and unbiased information among the family and professionals providing care for Chad.

SECTION III: PRACTICING FOR NCLEX

Activity F **CHOOSE THE BEST ANSWER.**

1. **Answer: a**
   RATIONALE: The affective function of the family provides for the emotional support of its members through love, encouragement, intimacy, and acceptance.

2. **Answer: d**
   RATIONALE: The child is an integral entity within the family; therefore, the focus of pediatric nursing is on the child and the family. The philosophy of care that has been adopted in pediatric healthcare is aptly called *family-centered care*. The child cannot be viewed as separate and apart from the group of individuals who play such an influential role in molding the child's behavior, emotions, and understanding of the world.

3. **Answer: b**
   RATIONALE: Despite the ongoing validation of the importance of family-centered care, actualizing family-centered care practices remains problematic. Technology, economic trends toward downsizing services and staffing, and the presence of a more culturally diverse population of patients are challenges to implementing family-centered care. Additionally, Newton (2000) identified family role

stress, negotiation failures, and power struggles as issues that affect the collaborative relationship between the family and the healthcare providers, and often impede family-centered care.

4. **Answer: c**
   RATIONALE: The socialization and social placement function is met when adult members take the responsibility of raising the children to be functional members of society. This occurs through effective parenting, education, and instillation of the family's culture, values, and religion. Parental involvement in the child's school and education has been associated with both better academic performance and improved social maturity.

5. **Answer: b**
   RATIONALE: The U.S. Census defines family as a group of two or more persons related by blood, marriage, or adoption who are residing together. Bozett (1987) defines family as whomever the patient says it is. The Institute for Family-Centered Care defines family as two or more persons who are related in any way—biologically, legally, or emotionally; Hanson defines family as two or more individuals who depend on one another for emotional, physical, and economic support.

6. **Answer: a**
   RATIONALE: Family-centered care is based on the premise that a positive adjustment to a child's level of health and well-being requires the involvement of the whole family (Lewandowski & Tesler, 2003; Shelton & Stepanek, 1995). Technology, economic trends toward downsizing services and staffing, and the presence of a more culturally diverse population of patients are challenges to implementing family-centered care.

7. **Answer: c**
   RATIONALE: Strategies to enhance family-centered care include encouraging family visiting in the postanesthesia room, changing visiting policies to promote the presence of the family at the bedside, involving parents in playroom activities, and incorporating the family in interdisciplinary conferences regarding the child's care.

8. **Answer: c**
   RATIONALE: A medical home is more than a building, house or hospital, or a specific healthcare team the person sees on a regular basis. The concept of a medical home is also an approach to providing healthcare services in a high-quality and cost-effective manner (Sobel & Healy, 2001).

9. **Answer: a**
   RATIONALE: In the family systems approach, the system is defined as a goal-directed unit made up of interdependent, interacting parts that endure over a period of time (Friedman, Bowden & Jones, 2003), and may be open or closed.

10. **Answer: c**
    RATIONALE: Nurses can use developmental theory to determine the types of stressors a family may be

facing at each developmental stage. In this case, anticipatory guidance can be given to the family to help them accommodate the needs of their adolescents into their family routines and rules.

Activity G CHOOSE ALL ANSWERS THAT APPLY.

1. **Answer: b, c, f**
   RATIONALE: Family-centered care involves incorporating into policy and practice the recognition that the family is the constant in a child's life, whereas the service systems and support personnel within those systems fluctuate, exchanging complete and unbiased information among families and professionals in a supportive manner at all times; incorporating into policy and practice the recognition and honoring of cultural diversity, strengths, and individuality; and encouraging and facilitating family-to-family support and networking.

2. **Answer: a, c, d, f**
   RATIONALE: The functional goal of the system is to ensure survival, continuity, and growth of its components (Friedman, Bowden & Jones, 2003). The open system depends on the interactions with the surrounding environment to achieve growth and change. As a unit, the family has boundaries that separate it from other systems. The family unit belongs to the many other systems that impinge on its boundaries. The family that has little exchange with the environment is one that resists change. A closed-unit family depends on edict and law and order, and operates through force, both physical and psychological.

3. **Answer: a, d**
   RATIONALE: Duvall (1962) was among the first to divide the family life cycle into eight stages with developmental tasks at each stage. These stages were based on the criteria of (1) major change in family size, (2) the developmental stage of the oldest child, and (3) the work status of the primary wage earner.

Activity H FILL IN THE BLANKS.

1. **Answer:** Communal family
   RATIONALE: People join communes to be surrounded by individuals who share common beliefs and practices; in many cases, these are religious beliefs. Principles that guide communal living include collective ownership; the absence of private property accumulation by individual members; and the collective responsibility for all material, cultural, educational, and health needs of the family.

2. **Answer:** Family
   RATIONALE: Family roles and family functions are closely related. Roles are the set of behaviors of an occupant of a particular social position. The family determines the role each family member should play to carry out the functions of the family.

CHAPTER 2

SECTION I: ASSESSING YOUR UNDERSTANDING

Activity A FILL IN THE BLANKS.

1. Advocate
2. Case manager
3. Health Insurance Portability and Accountability Act (HIPPA)
4. Needs assessments
5. Institutional Ethics Committee (IEC)
6. Informed consent

Activity B MATCH THE TERMS IN COLUMN A WITH THE PROPER DEFINITION LISTED IN COLUMN B.

1. d	2. f	3. c	4. g	5. e
6. a	7. b	8. i	9. h	

Activity C BRIEFLY ANSWER THE FOLLOWING.

1. A variety of strategies exist to improve child health, including
   - Seeking additional funding for key programs so that they can serve more children
   - Creating healthier and more supportive communities
   - Directing families to services, and teaching and supporting them as they advocate for themselves and their children

2. Opportunities to work in the community are available through public health agencies, hospitals, and community-based programs.

3. The family is the basic system in which health behavior and care are organized, secured, and performed. In most families, the parents or guardians, as advocates for their child, provide health promotion and health prevention care, as well as primary management of care when the child is sick. Parents and guardians also have the prime responsibility for initiating and coordinating services rendered by health professionals.

4. Communities can help improve the health of children and families by ensuring that resources are available, appropriate, and accessible. Likewise, for families of children with special healthcare needs, communities should ensure access to community activities and resources, and nurture the children's participation in them.

5. Communities should offer support to children and their families through tangible services such as self-help groups, counseling, food banks, and homeless shelters.

6. Head Start is a child development program aimed at preparing low-income preschoolers for school entry by including child development, school readiness, health, nutrition, and links to other social services in its program focus.

SECTION II: APPLYING YOUR KNOWLEDGE

Activity D **CONSIDER THIS SCENARIO AND ANSWER THE QUESTIONS.**

1. The nurse should act as a child advocate for this family and help them access programs that are available to them within the community. The nurse should also encourage Rupa to advocate for her child and herself, take responsibility for using these resources, and follow up when referrals have been offered to them. The nurse should act as a case manager for the family by determining their strengths and weaknesses, establishing goals, and developing a plan of care that explicitly states who will do what and when, and specifying the person who will assume accountability for each action item.

2. The role of the family is to advocate for Ela, to provide health promotion, health prevention care, and primary management of care when the Ela is sick. As the mother, Rupa is also responsible for initiating and coordinating services rendered by health professionals.

3. Communities have the responsibility to develop strategies to enhance access to services that already exist or create new services as needs demand. Strategies may involve such ideas as providing free or low-cost local transportation, providing low-cost child care, or collocating services to make one or more programs available at the same site. Improving access may also involve working with individual programs to increase "family friendliness" with extended hours, bilingual or bicultural workers, printed materials in easy-to-read formats, and a clear and simplified application process. Nurses may participate in community planning meetings to develop strategies for providing services or they may become involved in seeking funding for proposals by writing grants or making presentations to community groups.

SECTION III: PRACTICING FOR NCLEX

Activity E **CHOOSE THE BEST ANSWER.**

1. **Answer: b**
   RATIONALE: The Keep Your Child/Yourself Safe and Sound (KySS) program and the Healthy Eating and Activity Together (HEAT) initiative are examples of nationally based work undertaken by National Association of Pediatric Nurse Practitioners (NAPNAP). These two initiatives focus on the nurses' role in the prevention and early identification of psychosocial morbidities and overweight respectively.

2. **Answer: b**
   RATIONALE: Pain medication is appropriate for children receiving palliative care. For children with terminal conditions, medical treatment should only be used if the benefits outweigh the burdens to the child undergoing such therapies. This includes interventions such as organ transplantation, ventilator

therapy, dialysis, and use of vasoactive medications that prolong life or alter substantially the expected progression toward death.

3. **Answer: d**
   RATIONALE: Seeking permission for a DNR order is an undeniable signal to the parent that the healthcare team believes further lifesaving measures are not in the best interests of the child. The nurse's role when this occurs is to remain empathetic, acknowledge the parents' feelings, and answer any questions they may have. A decision to withhold or withdraw Life Sustaining Medical Treatment (LSMT) does not imply that the primary intent is to hasten the child's death; basic care such as suctioning, oxygen administration, and medication administration must continue unless ordered otherwise.

4. **Answer: b**
   RATIONALE: Federal regulations specifically prohibit withholding medically beneficial treatment from newborns with disabilities, except under specified conditions: permanent unconsciousness, "futile" treatment, and "virtually futile" interventions that are excessively burdensome for the infant.

5. **Answer: d**
   RATIONALE: Innovative therapies vary widely from minor variations of existing methods, extension of existing methods to new indications, to completely novel technologies (National Health and Medical Research Council, 1999). They are defined as new and unproved interventions that are performed with no intent to gather new information, and have not yet been fully assessed for safety and/or efficacy.

6. **Answer: d**
   RATIONALE: In a research study, the participants may or may not have access to the findings and can ask questions at any time before, during, or after the study. They should know that what they are agreeing to participate in is research and not part of standard care, and that they will know who the investigator is and how to contact him or her.

7. **Answer: c**
   RATIONALE: Qualifications for Medicaid include

   - All children born after September 30, 1993, with family incomes up to 100% of the federal poverty level
   - Children in federally assisted foster care and adoption placements
   - All pregnant women, infants, and children younger than 6 years of age with family income up to 133% of the federal poverty level whose resources do not exceed state-set limits
   - All infants born to Medicaid-enrolled women, for up to 1 year (no separate application required)

8. **Answer: b**
   RATIONALE: The goals of the MCH Block Grant Funds include providing access to quality maternal and child health services for mothers and children

with low income or limited availability to services; to provide prenatal, delivery, and postpartum care to at-risk women; to increase the number of children appropriately immunized; and to provide rehabilitation services for blind and disabled individuals younger than age 16 years receiving benefits under Title XVI.

9. **Answer: c**
   RATIONALE: Beneficence implies doing "good" and avoiding harm, and requires weighing the benefits and risks associated with participation in a study. Confidentiality refers to safeguarding the subject's identity. Justice focuses on the distribution of burden and benefits among the population of interest, and respect requires that the subject is able to independently and autonomously volunteer to participate in a study.

10. **Answer: a**
    RATIONALE: The Special Supplemental Food Program for Women, Infants and Children (WIC) provides nutritious food, health education, and links to healthcare resources to pregnant and lactating women, infants younger than age 1 year, and children up to age 5 years who are at risk for nutritional problems

Activity F **CHOOSE ALL ANSWERS THAT APPLY.**

1. **Answer: a, b, e, f**
   RATIONALE: Healthy People 2010: National Health Promotion and Disease Prevention Objectives for the Year 2010 is a key national initiative that has identified areas that need improvement and provides benchmarks to indicate success. Areas identified include immunization rates; injury and violence prevention; maternal, infant, and child care; and physical activity and fitness.

2. **Answer: a, c, d**
   RATIONALE: Adults have the right to self-determination for medical care after consultation with a physician or other healthcare provider. Until children reach the age of majority, which varies from state to state, or are legally emancipated, they lack the legal empowerment to make medical decisions on their own. Consent must be voluntary and based upon shared information about the risks and benefits of the treatment. The parent must understand the information and be cognitively and mentally competent to make the decision. Parents do not have the sole right to decide whether their decision is not in the child's best interest, and the child does not have the sole right to dissent if the intervention is deemed essential to his or her welfare.

Activity G **FILL IN THE BLANKS.**

1. Medicaid
2. Title V
3. Temporary Assistance for Needy Families

CHAPTER 3

SECTION I: ASSESSING YOUR UNDERSTANDING

Activity A **FILL IN THE BLANKS.**

1. Growth
2. Development
3. Teratogens
4. Predictable
5. Heredity
6. Operant
7. Surveillance
8. Cephalocaudal
9. Eighth
10. Extrusion
11. Temperament

Activity B **MATCH THE THEORISTS IN COLUMN A WITH THE EXAMPLES LISTED IN COLUMN B.**

1. c   2. d   3. g   4. a   5. h
6. i   7. b   8. f   9. j   10. i

Activity C **WRITE THE CORRECT SEQUENCE FOR CEPHALOCAUDAL GROSS MOTOR DEVELOPMENT IN THE BOXES.**

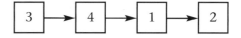

Activity D **BRIEFLY ANSWER THE FOLLOWING.**

1. a. Lack of adequate food intake to provide the protein and caloric needs of the body
   b. Social and cultural differences in food habits
   c. Widespread ease and availability of highly processed and often nutritionally inadequate foods
   d. Lack of adequate nutrition education in schools and in the home
   e. Complacency regarding food habits
   f. Overeating of foods that do not meet the needs of the body
   g. The presence of disease or illness that interferes with the ingestion, digestion, and absorption of food and/or that causes higher nutritional needs
   h. Failure to adjust nutritional intake based on changing levels of activity and rest, and on periods of higher metabolic demands (e.g., puberty)

2. Environmental factors are the psychological, social, and ecologic influences that affect the child's development. Factors such as parenting practices, interactions with peers, and frequent hospitalizations are examples of the psychological and social factors that influence individual development. Exposure to hazardous agents and nutritional intake are examples of ecologic factors that affect development.

Development of teeth and bones can be affected by the child's access to calcium and amount of fluoride in the drinking water. Ongoing research aims to analyze the ways in which nature (represented by genetics and heredity) combines with nurture (represented by a person's environment) to produce a given outcome. Four examples of environmental factors with examples include the following:

a. Pharmaceutical teratogens such as alcohol can cause fetal alcohol syndrome, and small-for-gestational-age newborn.

b. Infectious teratogens such as rubella virus can cause deafness, congenital heart disease, microcephaly, hepatosplenomegaly, mental retardation, and fetal death.

c. Family influences such as violence in the home can cause the child physical and emotional trauma.

d. Community/environmental influences such as secondhand smoke can cause premature death and disease in children as well as increased risk of sudden infant death syndrome (SIDS), acute respiratory problems, ear infections, and more severe asthma.

3. a. Stage 1 is Punishment and Obedience Orientation and includes ages 5 to 8. Children at this age will avoid breaking rules to avoid punishment.

b. Stage 2 is Instrumental Relativist Orientation and includes ages 7 to 10. Right actions satisfy the child's own needs and sometimes the needs of others. The child desires to serve one's own interests. Helping others incurs a debt to be collected later.

c. Stage 3 is Interpersonal Concordance of "Good Boy–Nice Girl" Orientation and includes ages 10 to 12. Good behavior is what pleases or helps others and is approved by them. Children have the need to see themselves as a good person and need to gain approval of others.

d. Stage 4 is the Law and Order Orientation and includes ages 12 to 25. Belief in the Golden Rule and a desire to maintain rules and follow authority to support stereotypical good behavior are the reasons for the moral actions.

e. Stage 5 is the Social Contract Legalistic Orientation and includes ages 25 to 35 (if reached). During this stage, the person is aware that people hold a variety of values and opinions even though there are also rights and rules that have been constitutionally and democratically agreed on. The reasoning for the moral action is obligation to law because of one's social contract with society, and good is done because it serves the greatest number of people.

f. Stage 6 is the Universal Ethical Principle Orientation and includes ages 25 to 35 (if reached). The moral outlook includes self-chosen ethical principles based on abstract principles that are the foundation for action. Laws or social agreements are considered valid because they are consistent with one's ethical principles. The moral reasoning includes a belief and commitment to the validity of universal moral principles. There is a desire to uphold abstract principles that define right behavior for self. When unjust laws conflict with the broad moral principles, the laws may be broken.

4. There are four developmental considerations for hearing based on age.

a. Ages from birth to 3 months:
- The infant should startle to loud noises, random activity diminishes with sounds, and environmental sounds will waken the sleeping infant.
- The infant may have fluid or mucous in the Eustachian tube or vernix caseosa in the external ear canal. These conditions resolve quickly. Infants who do not startle to loud noises should be further evaluated for hearing loss and further assessed for causes. The cause of congenital hearing loss could be infections in utero, anomalies, and genetic. Hearing loss is greater in premature children.

b. Three to 4 months:
- The infant should turn toward the sound of the mother's voice. The infant begins to coo and gurgles in response to speech, and is quieted by pleasant sounds (voice or music).
- Infants who do not respond with these behaviors may have the problems undiagnosed in the 0- to 3-month age group and should be further evaluated.

c. Five to 9 months:

Mimics sounds and responds differently to angry and pleasant voices. The infant enjoys musical toys and reacts to soft sounds as whispers.

d. Twelve to 15 months:
- The child responds when his name is called and vocally will imitate sounds. Child should have five to eight words by this age.
- Children who do not have these hearing behaviors or who do not progress with their language skills could have permanent partial hearing loss associated with bacterial meningitis, severe otitis media, and certain infectious diseases (mumps, measles, Epstein-Barr virus), the use of ototoxic drugs, and head trauma. These children would need evaluation because hearing is crucial especially early in childhood for the development of language.

5. a. The individuality of a child's growth and development is highly influenced by factors such as heredity, the environment, nutrition, sensory stimulation, and affection.

b. Growth is systematic and occurs in a sequential pattern.

c. Although growth is a systematic process, body systems vary in their rates of development.

d. When evaluating a child's growth, it is important to assess the child's patterns of growth over several months or years, rather than base an entire assessment on a single evaluation of the child at a particular time.

e. The terms *normal* or *average* have been used to describe the predictable patterns of growth and development that have been studied and are known to occur within a certain time frame. From this normal or average pattern, each child can be viewed as a variation of the theme.

f. The child's development of skills and functions proceeds from the simple to the complex and from the general to the specific.

g. Development progresses in a head-to-toe, or cephalocaudal fashion, and in a proximal–distal, or midline to the periphery, progression.

h. As the child grows and matures, some critical periods are known to exist. These time periods refer to points during which the individual is highly sensitive or ready for certain actions.

i. Each individual's growth and development trajectory, however, is influenced by environmental factors such as nutrition and sensory stimulation. If these environmental factors are either strongly negative or positive, effects on child's growth and development patterns may be altered.

j. All humans have an inherent desire to learn and grow. Abraham Maslow called this *self-actualization*; Carl Rogers called it *directional growth*.

SECTION II: APPLYING YOUR KNOWLEDGE
Activity E CONSIDER THE SCENARIO AND ANSWER THE QUESTIONS.

1. The cognitive stage of development Emily's behavior demonstrates is preconceptual stage 1 (2–4 years) within the preoperational stage (2–7 years).

2. The nurse should share with the mother that the behavior Emily displays is expected behavior for a 2-year-old. A 2-year-old is egocentric and is centered on self. At this age, children are not able to see

things from another's perspective. Children in this stage of development are unaware of others feeling and experiences. Emily satisfies her own needs by taking toys she wants away from others without any awareness of the other child's feelings. As Emily grows and develops, she will learn to share. The mother can help Emily give the toy back while redirecting Emily to another desirable toy. Parallel play with children side by side, but with little interaction between them, occurs in this age group.

SECTION III: PRACTICING FOR NCLEX
Activity F ANSWER THE FOLLOWING QUESTIONS.

1. **Answer: d**
RATIONALE: Ninety-five percent of children walk independently by 18 months. Further assessment is necessary to confirm or rule out developmental delay.

2. **Answer: c**
RATIONALE: By 8 months of age, the infant can sit upright for long periods of time. Between 5 and 6 months of age, the spinal column has straightened enough and head control is sufficient to allow the infant to sit. The child can also easily change from a lying to a sitting position and vice versa.

3. **Answer: d**
RATIONALE: At 4 years of age the child can hop, and walk down the stairs on alternating feet. By 5 years the child has also learned to skip, demonstrating simple movements to the more complex skip. The terms *normal* or *average* have been used to describe the predictable patterns of growth and development that have been studied and are known to occur within a certain time frame. Within the 5-year-old time frame, these abilities are expected to be accomplished.

4. **Answer: b**
RATIONALE: Maslow is considered a humanistic theorist. All people desire to become all that they are capable of being. Maslow presents a hierarchical theory in which basic needs are met first and then the person moves to higher levels of achievement to self-actualization. Emphasis is on the here and now to move forward.

5. **Answer: a**
RATIONALE: Operant conditioning holds that behaviors are repeated or are reduced in frequency based on the environmental consequences of reinforcement or punishment. When the child's

behavior is followed by a negative or positive reinforcer, it decreases or increases the chances of the behavior being repeated.

6. **Answer: c**
   RATIONALE: Children at this age need the mother to be present and close for a sense of security. The child is in stage 2, preconceptual or intuitive stage (4–7 years), and prelogical reasoning appears. Children need a simple explanation and the unpleasant experience to be completed quickly. The child can concentrate on one characteristic of an object at a time, so a syringe to handle will divert her and decrease her anticipation and anxiety. The syringe can also be used for her to play giving injection to a doll.

7. **Answer: a**
   RATIONALE: Infants at this age are teething and the infant can bite down on the block for comfort. The infant can pick up the block and transfer it to the other hand and even hand the block back and forth to an adult. All other objects listed are beyond the developmental level of an infant of 9 months.

8. **Answer: d**
   RATIONALE: The child is walking as expected for his age and the length of time he has been walking. Children, when beginning to walk, have a wide base of support and sometimes stumble. Children will become more balanced, become more upright, and will assume a narrow base of support after walking 19 months from the initiation of walking.

9. **Answer: b**
   RATIONALE: The flexed position would be expected because newborns assume this position in utero. Arms and legs are flexed and when extended the extremities return to the flexed position. This is characteristic of term infants. The premature infant will have less flexion of the extremities, depending on the gestational age at birth.

10. **Answer: c**
    RATIONALE: Transient strabismus is normal in newborns and will resolve within the first couple of months. Ethnicity does not influence the transient strabismus in newborns.

11. **Answer: a**
    RATIONALE: Eilind describes this as adolescent egocentric thought processes. Adolescents believe they are at the center of attention and all eyes are focused on them. The term used is *superself-consciousness*. Adolescents are focused on their own actions, spend little time concerned about others, and think they are more special.

12. **Answer: b**
    RATIONALE: The Denver II is among one of the most commonly used developmental screening instruments. The screening tool is administered by trained healthcare personnel and is an overall assessment of development administered in 15 to 20 minutes. A parent-answered prescreening form is also available.

13. **Answer: d**
    RATIONALE: According to Piaget, a 17-year-old can logically manipulate abstract and unobservable concepts. The understanding of the surgery for this age group is best served with an explanation and opportunity to ask questions. Kohlberg's stage 4, Law and Order Orientation, can be reinforced by respecting the adolescent and taking time for questions and clarification.

14. **Answer: b**
    RATIONALE: Visual cues such as gestures like waving bye-bye are an important element to convey expressive meaning. Visual language helps the child develop auditory expressive and auditory receptive language.

15. **Answer: b**
    RATIONALE: Girls are generally more advanced than boys in verbal acquisition. During early childhood, girls demonstrate advanced development of the left cerebral hemisphere—the speech center of the brain.

16. **Answer:** Weight: 5×26 lb $= 130$ lb Height: 2×32 in $= 64$ in or 5 ft 4 in
    RATIONALE: These formulas are a general guide for estimating expected adult stature using the weight and height of an 18-month-old child.

17. **Answer: c**
    RATIONALE: The child's race and ethnicity influence patterns of growth and development in obvious and subtle ways.

18. **Answer: d**
    RATIONALE: The child at this stage of growth and development believes bad things happen because of their behavior. The child views the accident as a result of his being bad according to stages of faith development.

19. **Answer: a, b, e, f**

CHAPTER 4

SECTION I: ASSESSING YOUR UNDERSTANDING

Activity A MATCH THE TERM IN COLUMN A WITH THE PROPER DEFINITION IN COLUMN B.

1. c   **2.** b   **3.** e   **4.** a   **5.** d

Activity B FILL IN THE BLANKS.

1. Neck
2. 12
3. 6
4. Car seat
5. Childproofing

Activity C BRIEFLY ANSWER THE FOLLOWING.

1. R: Regulating the infant's state, preventing overarousal, calms the infant; E: Environmental cues, such as light and dark, noise and quiet, help synchronize the infant's behavior; S: Structure and repetition makes events reassuringly predictable for the infant; T: Touch soothes the child and diminishes stimulation.

2. Eye-to-eye contact, physical contact, and communication.
3. Expressed breast milk can be stored in the refrigerator for up to 8 days; prepared formula, 24 hours.
4. Propping increases the risk of aspiration of the formula and otitis media.

SECTION II: APPLYING YOUR KNOWLEDGE

Activity D CONSIDER THE SCENARIO AND ANSWER THE QUESTIONS.

1. The nurse should calmly approach the mother and offer her encouraging words and verbal assistance, resisting any temptation to take over. Provide reassurance that this is a learning period for both the new mother and the infant. Take the time to help the mother complete the task. This will give the nurse an opportunity to build a trusting relationship with the mother and assess her needs and concerns, and to develop an individualized discharge teaching plan. It is encouraging that this new young mother is actively participating in her child's care and is having physical contact with the child.
2. Key questions would include the following:
   - Was this a planned or unexpected pregnancy?
   - Did she take any prenatal or parenting classes prior to childbirth?
   - Does she have any support at home such as friends, family, or a significant other?
   - Does she have any previous knowledge or experience caring for children?
   - Does she plan to breast-feed or bottle-feed?
   - What are her available resources, including housing, transportation, finances, and so forth?

   In addition, the nurse would want to look for mother–infant bonding and attachment. The nurse would look for certain identifiable behaviors, including eye-to-eye contact, physical contact, and communication, to indicate that attachment is occurring. The nurse should be concerned if the parent avoids eye contact and physical contact with the infant or if, when contact is unavoidable, the infant is not held close to the parent's body. The nurse also needs to assess the mother's level of comfort and her major concerns. If the nurse can put to rest any concerns the mother may have up front, the discharge teaching process will be more productive and progress smoothly.
3. Whenever possible, as much information as possible about the patient should be provided, both verbally and written. Many hospitals have discharge teaching videos that are provided to new mothers to view prior to discharge. The nurse should discuss the following in her discharge plan:

- Developmental milestones for neonates and infants, and state measures to enhance meeting these milestones.
- The needs of the infant related to hygiene, personal care, nutrition, elimination, and safety. Include instructions on how to give the child a bath, and how to provide oral and perineal care.
- How to select age-appropriate interventions to promote healthy personal and social development of the infant.
- When to schedule for well-baby checkups, the importance of the immunization schedule, and when to call or take the child to the doctor with an illness.
- How to take the infant's temperature, and the importance of hand washing and avoiding infections.
- How to select interventions to promote illness and injury prevention for the infant and the family.
- Health supervision of the infant includes healthcare visits at 1, 2, 4, 6, 9, and 12 months of age. Specific immunizations and diagnostic tests are scheduled for each healthcare visit, and the child is assessed to determine whether development is proceeding normally.
- Infant care includes attending to bathing and skin care needs. Special attention should be given to the child's safety during these activities, such as how to set the water heater temperature to avoid burns and never to leave the infant unattended in the tub.
- Gum and oral care is started soon after birth. Explain the pattern of teething and measures to decrease discomfort, such as Tylenol administration and cool compresses. Explain that there is associated irritability when a child is teething.
- With regard to sleep patterns, during the first month of life, the neonate sleeps 16 to 20 hours per day. Throughout the first year of life, this number will decrease to an average of 13.75 hours per day by 1 year of age.
- With regard to infant nutrition, current recommendations include breast-feeding exclusively for approximately the first 6 months and supporting breast-feeding for the first year of life.
- Breast- and bottle-feeding techniques must be learned.
- Introduce solid foods to the infant's diet at 4 to 6 months of age, based upon the infant's developmental readiness. Cereal products are the first solids to be introduced.
- With regard to elimination issues, the parent should expect 6 to 10 wet diapers per day. Stools of breast-fed infants differ in color, smell, and consistency from those of bottle-fed infants. As the child matures, elimination patterns will become more rhythmic and individualized.
- Temperament is the natural inborn style of behavior of each child. Environmental

stimulation of the child should be gauged toward the child's unique temperament and activity needs.

- The nurse should explain that the infant's parent(s) is responsible for providing an environment that is safe. Safety prevention measures must include crib safety, car safety, water safety, home safety, and toy safety.

SECTION III: PRACTICING FOR NCLEX

Activity E CHOOSE THE BEST ANSWER.

1. d   **2.** a   **3.** d   **4.** c   **5.** b
6. c   **7.** a

CHAPTER 5

SECTION I: ASSESSING YOUR UNDERSTANDING

Activity A MATCH THE TERMS IN COLUMN A WITH THE APPROPRIATE CONSIDERATIONS FROM COLUMN B.

1. d   **2.** a   **3.** e   **4.** c   **5.** b

Activity B FILL IN THE BLANKS.

1. Learning
2. Bedtime
3. Imagination
4. Dressing

Activity C BRIEFLY ANSWER THE FOLLOWING.

1. Night terrors occur during the early hours of sleep, and the child does not fully awaken nor rarely remembers the episode in the morning. Nightmares occur during the second half of the sleep period, and the child awakes, has trouble falling back to sleep, and usually remembers the episode in the morning.

With night terrors, the parents should ensure the child's safety, let them take their course, and not interact with the child. With nightmares, the parents should reassure the child that it was just a dream, comfort the child, and postpone talking about it until morning.

2. Sibling rivalry refers to the normal reaction of jealousy and resentment to someone new joining the family. Involvement in newborn care helps the toddler adapt better. Parents should not introduce a new developmental task at this time, but should spend extra time alone with the toddler.

3. Precautions include never giving small hard foods such as peanuts or hard candies. Even soft, small

foods, such as grapes, could be a hazard. Foods should be mashed or cut into small pieces to prevent choking, and the child should be sitting down for all snacks and mealtimes instead of being handed a snack and allowed to walk or run with it. Parents should provide age-appropriate foods, supervise snack and mealtimes, and teach proper eating behavior.

SECTION II: APPLYING YOUR KNOWLEDGE

Activity D CONSIDER THE SCENARIO AND ANSWER THE QUESTIONS.

1. Devon's desire to eat only macaroni and cheese is an example of a food jag. This is a period when a child will eat only a few foods, being very particular about food.

2. The nurse needs to explain food jags to the mother and that this is typical of toddlers and preschoolers. The nurse would then encourage Janice to avoid power struggles at mealtimes and inform her that it might take 10 to 15 attempts before a child will try a new food. When introducing a new food, have Janice encourage the child to taste it or combine a new food with a favorite one. Advise her that the child's initial refusal does not necessarily represent a permanent dislike of the food. Encourage her to offer it again in a few days and if the child is not forced to eat it, the child often will accept it. Also urge her not to negotiate what the child eats, reward the child with treats, or threaten punishment.

3. The nurse needs to explain to Janice that temper tantrums are a common way for young children to deal with frustrations associated with trying to assert their independence. In addition, Janice needs to know that breath holding does not cause permanent damage because as the oxygen level decreases and the carbon dioxide level increases, respiration is stimulated. A key component of dealing with temper tantrums involves remaining calm. Janice should be instructed to allow Devon to make frequent small choices within specified parameters and should be consistent in using the word *no*. If a temper tantrum occurs, Janice needs to ignore the behavior (but ensure Devon's safety), avoiding eye contact or interaction until the child has calmed down. Afterward, Janice should discuss his behavior with him in a calm, neutral tone and provide the child with ways to get "in control."

SECTION III: PRACTICING FOR NCLEX

Activity E CHOOSE THE BEST ANSWER.

1. d   **2.** b   **3.** a   **4.** b   **5.** a

CHAPTER 6

SECTION I: ASSESSING YOUR UNDERSTANDING

Activity A MATCH THE TERM IN COLUMN A WITH THE PHRASE IN COLUMN B.

1. c   **2.** g   **3.** h   **4.** a   **5.** e
6. b   **7.** d   **8.** f

Activity B MATCH THE TERM IN COLUMN A WITH THE PHRASE IN COLUMN B.

1. e   **2.** b   **3.** g   **4.** f   **5.** a
6. d   **7.** c   **8.** h

Activity C PLACE THE FOLLOWING STEPS IN THE PROPER ORDER.

1.
2.

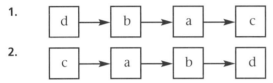

Activity D FILL IN THE BLANKS.

1. Collecting
2. Food pyramid
3. Television
4. Bedtime
5. Adults
6. Six
7. Self-esteem
8. School readiness

SECTION II: APPLYING YOUR KNOWLEDGE

Activity E BRIEFLY ANSWER THE FOLLOWING.

1. The "difficult" child is usually the child who is the most challenging to live with. The nurse needs to assist the parents in determining good strategies when dealing with the child. The nurse can coach the parents to remain neutral or objective during emotional situations and not to take the child's behavior personally. Teach the parents possible high-risk situations and strategies to deal with these situations effectively.

2. Parents often make a child stay in a time-out until he or she does what the parent wants done. This is incorrect. Instead, time-outs should be used to teach the child how to regain self-control and calm down. Other considerations for effective time-outs are as follows:

- It must be timed appropriately.
- Brief time-outs are more effective.
- The maximum duration should be 1 minute for each year of age.
- It should end as soon as the child is calm.

- Time-out does not need to occur only in the child's room.

3. Play activities are called the *work* of the child because they help the child to master new skills, manage relations with other children, and build self-confidence and self-esteem.

4. During middle childhood, making friends and sustaining those relationships is one of the most important social accomplishments. The child is able to form complex relationships, and communication has developed to a point that the child can share feelings with friends and family. The child may develop a "best friend" that usually complements them and they feel completely comfortable with that person.

Activity F CONSIDER THE SCENARIO AND ANSWER THE QUESTIONS.

1. Easton's behavior for his developmental age is normal. Preschoolers have fear of body mutilation and strong imaginations. Because Easton is in a new environment and has most likely never seen these people or taken this medication before this incidence, his imagination is probably running wild. He may even think that the medication will hurt him and make him have to stay at the hospital.

2. The hospitalized preschooler is a challenge for the healthcare staff. It is important to facilitate plan care that is developmentally appropriate and continues to build the child's self esteem.

- Magical thinking: Preschoolers interpret things literally and have vivid imaginations. For example, if a preschooler receives an IV or shot, he or she may believe that he or she may bleed to death.
- Fears: Loss of control and body mutilation
- Body mutilation: Preschoolers fear loss of limbs and mutilation
- Regression, loss of control: Often, as in toddlerhood, preschoolers may regress to previous behaviors.
- Interpret hospitalization as punishment: Preschoolers often believe that their hospitalization is a form of punishment or because they did something "bad."

3. Goal: Patient will actively participate in care and activities of daily living.
Interventions:

- Explain all procedures and interventions immediately before beginning.
- Allow the child to play with or handle equipment (within safety limits) to familiarize him- or herself with the unfamiliar.
- Give the child choices and allow him or her to make decisions.
- Give encouragement and positive feedback for good behavior.
- Offer a reward from the "toy chest" or sticker after the procedure is over.
- Assess child's home routine and stick to that schedule as much as possible.
- Listen and spend time with the child.

- Continue fostering learning new skills, assisting with activities of daily living, potty training, and so forth.
- Initiate age-appropriate play activities; this helps to master new skills and alleviate fears.

SECTION III: PRACTICING FOR NCLEX

Activity G **CHOOSE THE BEST ANSWER.**

1. **Answer: d**
   RATIONALE: Asking open-ended trigger questions are best when trying to elicit information from the parents regarding the preschooler's development. The other questions are more likely to generate a positive response from the parent even though they lack clear information about the expected milestone.

2. **Answer: d**
   RATIONALE: Feeding strikes are normal. It is best just to continue to offer a wide variety of foods without comment. Refusing to feed the child her desired foods, showing how you like the new food, or insisting she take a bite unnecessarily turn the dinner table into a battleground.

3. **Answer: c**
   RATIONALE: A child should be encouraged to establish a homework routine. Offer a quiet place with no distractions to help the child study. Keep family schedules, but show the child it is important to keep his or her routine as well.

4. **Answer: b**
   RATIONALE: The most important recommendation is to prepare as much as possible the night before and avoid rushing in the morning. Rushing tends to cause stress for the parents, and the child feels the tension and may be upset when the parent leaves, thinking he or she did something wrong. The other suggestions can all be helpful, but establishing a routine and avoiding rushing is the most important.

5. **Answer: a**
   RATIONALE: By the age of 5 years, most preschoolers can hold their pencil like an adult. The other responses indicate that the girl has achieved many of her milestones involving gross motor skills. The nurse should follow up with more trigger questions that would elicit responses about the girl's fine motor skills.

6. **Answer: a**
   RATIONALE: Parents should avoid labeling a child a *picky eater*. Initial refusal of a new food does not always represent a permanent dislike. Children have personal likes and dislikes as all individuals do, but they may change. The nurse should simply remind the mother to continue offering a wide variety of foods and avoid labeling one son as *picky*.

7. **Answer: c**
   RATIONALE: The mother needs a plan to get this situation back under control. Encouraging the mother to stop feeding her son separately and to begin serving him the same food as the rest of the family are parts of the plan. There may be other dynamics contributing to this problem that can be uncovered with a little probing. Telling the mother she needs to quit pampering the child, does not teach.

8. **Answer: c**
   RATIONALE: Many variations exist regarding when children master various cognitive, linguistic, and fine and gross motor skills. Parents should not be discouraged or concerned because their child is not reading or coloring within the lines like another child of the same age. Although the nurse is confident that the boy has consistently been achieving developmental milestones, the mother is still concerned. A Denver Developmental Screening test would be a concrete way to assess the child's skills and provide reassurance that the boy is performing within the normal range for his age. The other responses have already proved ineffective and the mother needs additional reassurance.

9. **Answer: d**
   RATIONALE: Preschoolers need 10 to 11 hours of sleep per day. It is important to establish a consistent, relaxing bedtime routine that the girl will enjoy. Engaging in fun games before bedtime should be avoided. Simply insisting that the girl go to bed is likely to be ineffective. The girl needs to learn how to fall asleep rather than staying up with her brothers until she is exhausted.

10. **Answer: a**
    RATIONALE: The best response is offering developmentally appropriate choices for the child while validating the girl's intelligence. Telling the mother that standardized testing is the only way to measure giftedness is unhelpful and does not teach. The other responses are accurate, but are less tactful and do not offer appropriate alternatives.

CHAPTER 7

SECTION I: ASSESSING YOUR UNDERSTANDING

Activity A **MATCH THE DESCRIPTION IN COLUMN A WITH THE APPROPRIATE ANSWER IN COLUMN B.**

1. f   **2.** c   **3.** d   **4.** e   **5.** a
6. b

Activity B **MATCH THE TYPE OF DEVELOPMENTAL MILESTONE IN COLUMN A WITH THE DESCRIPTION OF THE MILESTONE IN COLUMN B.**

1. c   **2.** d   **3.** e   **4.** a   **5.** b

Activity C PLACE THE FOLLOWING DEVELOPMENTAL MILESTONES IN THE PROPER SEQUENCE.

Answers:

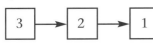

Activity D FILL IN THE BLANKS.

1. Puberty
2. Menarche
3. Branding
4. Body modification surgery
5. Folate
6. Strength training
7. Condoms
8. Abstinence

SECTION II: APPLYING YOUR KNOWLEDGE

Activity E BRIEFLY ANSWER THE FOLLOWING.

1. Answers:
   - Balance calorie intake with physical activity.
   - Ensure daily physical activity lasts 60 minutes or longer.
   - Eat fruits and vegetables liberally, and limit juice intake.
   - Use vegetable oils and margarines low in saturated fats and trans fatty acids.
   - Eat whole-grain products.
   - Reduce intake of sugar-sweetened beverages and foods.
   - Drink nonfat or low-fat milk.
   - Reduce salt intake.
   - Eat more legumes and tofu in stead of meats.
   - Limit snacking during sedentary activity.
   - Take a supplemental daily vitamin.

2. Answers:
   - Fosters a feeling of accomplishment
   - Reduces the risk of certain diseases
   - Promotes mental health
   - Assists in achieving healthy body weight and composition, reducing the risk of obesity
   - Promotes a healthy lifestyle throughout life

3. Answer: Early initiation is most likely to occur in children with learning problems or low academic attainment, children with behavioral or emotional problems (including mental health and substance abuse), children from low-income families, victims of physical and sexual abuse, and children in families with marital discord and low levels of parental supervision.

Activity F CONSIDER THE SCENARIO AND ANSWER THE QUESTIONS.

1. Remind the mother that the influences of television and movies leads many teenagers to have an idealized body image or misinformation about sex. Information is provided in school education courses, but many teenagers need answers about issues that they do not want to discuss in school. Encourage the mother as well as the father to share their feelings and values regarding sexual activity. Encourage them not to shy away from these discussions. Promote open lines of communication between the parents and teens. Encourage parents to listen to, rather than lecture, the teen.

2. Explain to Ellie's mom that early initiation of sexual activity can be the result of many factors, but that it is more commonly associated in children with learning disabilities, children with low academic attainment, and children with behavioral and emotional issues. Early sexual initiation is seen in children from low-income families, victims of physical and sexual abuse, children in families with marital discord, and children that are from families with decreased parental supervision.

3. There are many essentials that need to be discussed, the discussion should begin with her body and the function of her body's organs. She will need to become aware of how her sexuality affects and is tied to her body image. She should discuss the other gender's sexuality and sexual organs. She will need to discover the normalcy of sexual feelings. She will need to be taught about the act of sex. She will need to develop an understanding of sexual orientation. Discuss safe sex, pregnancy, and sexually transmitted diseases. Discuss sexual exploitation, sexual abuse, and emotional abuse.

SECTION III: PRACTICING FOR NCLEX

Activity G CHOOSE THE BEST ANSWER.

1. **Answer: d**
   RATIONALE: Asking open-ended trigger questions are best when trying to elicit information from the parents regarding the child's development. The other questions are more likely to generate a positive response from the parent even though they lack clear information about the expected milestone.

2. **Answer: d**
   RATIONALE: A compromise is the best choice for a 12-year-old. Limit the number of days the girl purchases school lunches and enlist her to prepare her own school lunch. Allowing children to prepare their own school lunches encourages them to make choices of foods that they will eat and not discard or trade. Advising the mother to let the girl make her own food choices does not address the mother's concerns. Refusing to let the girl purchase lunches does not promote compromise.

3. **Answer: a**
   RATIONALE: Spontaneous erections and nocturnal seminal emissions do not mean that the child is sexually active or is having overactive sexual thoughts. Parents need to be instructed that these

occurrences are spontaneous and that the child is not doing anything to cause them.

4. **Answer: a**
   RATIONALE: A primary goal of developmental surveillance is to promote adolescent self-advocacy—that is, to assist the adolescent in seeking out, evaluating, and using information to promote his or her health. Teaching the adolescent to ask for information and make decisions about his or her own care, and encouraging health promotion activities provides the adolescent with self advocacy. Adolescents report that they want to receive healthcare from competent professionals who demonstrate warmth and compassion. They want to receive care from professionals who communicate in a straightforward, understandable fashion. Providing the adolescent with respect and showing compassion are likely to help develop a strong relationship with the adolescent.

5. **Answer: b**
   RATIONALE: These parties are on the rise, and the removal of body hair—localized or all over the body—has increased. There is an increase in folliculitis caused by *Staphylococcus aureus*. Blood-born pathogens and infectious agents can be transferred when shaving supplies are shared. Shaving can cause irritation in any area. Discuss safe shaving practices with adolescents to ensure that the adolescent will seek medical attention if a rash does occur.

6. **Answer: b**
   RATIONALE: A quick way to assess fat intake is to ask the girl to perform a food recall for the past 24 hours. Asking whether the girl watches the amount of fat or whether she eats low-fat or fat-free foods is likely to elicit only a yes or no response. Inquiring about the amount of fat grams is inappropriate for a 14-year-old and is less informative than a food recall.

7. **Answer: b**
   RATIONALE: The nurse should first assess the girl's knowledge related to calcium intake and ask about other sources of calcium in her diet besides milk. Suggesting chocolate milk might be a helpful alternative to white milk, but only after they evaluate the other sources of calcium in the girl's diet. Asking the girl whether she thinks she is getting enough calcium is unhelpful and does not teach. Asking what the girl has on her cereal in the morning is unhelpful and does not open a dialogue about calcium sources.

8. **Answer: c**
   RATIONALE: Assessing the patient's sleep patterns for several weeks gives the healthcare provider the information needed to plot the trend in sleep patterns to determine whether there is a problem. Family history of insomnia does not affect the patient. Asking the patient the amount of sleep acquired in one night does not give the healthcare provider the

information needed to make a clinical judgment. Interrupted sleep would affect the teenage, but this can also be caused by an underlying condition and may lead to further investigation.

CHAPTER 8

SECTION I: ASSESSING YOUR UNDERSTANDING

Activity A MATCH THE AUSCULATORY SITE IN COLUMN A WITH THE DESCRIPTION IN COLUMN B.

1. c   **2.** a   **3.** d   **4.** b   **5.** e

Activity B MATCH THE DEEP TENDON REFLEX IN COLUMN A WITH THE ASSOCIATED NORMAL FINDING IN COLUMN B.

1. e   **2.** a   **3.** d   **4.** c   **5.** b

Activity C FILL IN THE BLANKS.

1. Coloboma
2. Anaphylactic
3. Confidential
4. Ecchymosis
5. Apical

SECTION II: APPLYING YOUR KNOWLEDGE

Activity D CONSIDER THE SCENARIO AND ANSWER THE QUESTIONS.

1. The nurse would assess the typical infant reflexes for Michael. Michael would most likely demonstrate a positive Babinski reflex which may be present up to 24 months of age. The dancing/stepping and gallant reflexes should not be present (these typically disappears by 4 to 8 weeks of age). The rooting, Moro, asymmetric tonic neck, sucking, and extrusion reflexes also should be absent (persistence beyond the age of 4 months is abnormal). Michael may still be exhibiting the palmar grasp reflex (considered abnormal if it persists beyond 10 months), but this should be beginning to disappear. In addition, Michael should exhibit the neck righting reflex and parachute reflex.

2. Anthropometric measurements for Michael would include height, weight and head circumference; for Jaron, these would include just height and weight. For Michael, height measurement is best done by placing the vertex of his head at the top of a flat measuring board and the soles of the feet firmly against the footboard. For Jaron, a wall-mounted stadiometer provides the most accurate standing height measurement. Place the movable measuring rod on the topmost part of the child's head while he or she is standing without shoes and with the

heels, buttocks, and shoulders just touching the wall. Instruct the child to look straight ahead without tilting the head. Michael would be weighed on an infant scale, whereas Jaron would be weighed using a stand-up scale. Michael's head circumference would be measured by wrapping a paper tape measure around the maximum occipitofrontal circumference. Measuring Jaron's head circumference would not be necessary.

3. To calculate Jaron's body mass index, the nurse would take Jaron's weight in pounds divided by his height in inches squared and then multiply by 703:

$$40/(42 \times 42) \times 703 = 15.99$$

Alternatively, the nurse could take Jaron's weight in kilograms (40 lbs = 18.2 kg) divide it by his height in centimeters (42 inches = 106.7 cm) squared and then multiply it by 10,000.

$$18.2 \text{ kg}/(106.7 \times 106.7) \times 10,000 = 15.94$$

4. As a 6-month-old, Michael could receive a dose of Hepatitis B vaccine (HepB) anywhere from 6 to 18 months of age. He would need a final dose of rotavirus vaccine by age 8 months. He would be scheduled to receive his third dose of DTaP at 6 months. If Michael received the PRP-OMP form of the Hib vaccine, a dose at age 6 months would not be needed. A dose of pneumococcal vaccine is typically given at age 6 months. Michael can receive his yearly influenza vaccine starting at age 6 months and inactivated poliovirus vaccine anywhere from 6 months to 18 months of age.

Jaron, who is 4 years old could receive his final dose of DTaP and inactivated poliovirus vaccine from ages 4 to 6 years. He would also receive his second dose of MMR and varicella between the ages of 4 to 6 years. In addition, Jaron should receive a yearly influenza vaccine if he hasn't had one as of yet.

SECTION III: PRACTICING FOR NCLEX
Activity E CHOOSE THE BEST ANSWER.
1. a **2.** c **3.** b **4.** a **5.** d
6. b **7.** d **8.** c

CHAPTER 9

SECTION I: ASSESSING YOUR UNDERSTANDING
Activity A FILL IN THE BLANKS.
1. Pharmacokinetics
2. Body surface area
3. Pharmacodynamics
4. Oral
5. Approach

6. Military
7. Verbal
8. Ice pop

Activity B MATCH THE DEVELOPMENTAL LEVEL OF THE CHILD IN COLUMN A WITH PROPER MEDICATION ADMINISTRATION APPROACH IN COLUMN B.
1. c **2.** d **3.** a **4.** b

Activity C WRITE THE CORRECT SEQUENCE OF MEDICATION ADMINISTRATION IN THE BOXES PROVIDED.

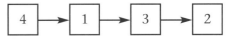

Activity D WRITE THE CORRECT SEQUENCE OF THE ADMINISTRATION OF A TOPICAL MEDICATION.

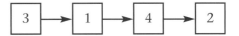

Activity E BRIEFLY ANSWER THE FOLLOWING.

1. The six rights of medication administration include
   - The right medication: Know the medication to be administered, and its indication for use, action, contraindications, and side effects. Understand the connection between the patient's condition, illness, or disease and the use of a particular medication. Select the correct medication from the patient's medication drawer or from medications sent to the unit from the pharmacy. Verify the medication label with the patient's medication administration record.
   - The right dose: Pediatric dosages are calculated based on weight in kilograms or BSA. Adult dose reference ranges, rather than kilogram dosing, may be used in children who weigh more than 50 kg. Always double-check math calculations and compare calculations with the actual order to verify that it is within the recommended range.
   - The right patient: All children who have been admitted to a healthcare facility should be identified by an identification band attached to their body and not according to the bed they are in.
   - The right route: The route of administration affects the absorption, effectiveness, and the speed of action of medications.
   - The right time: Medications given at the wrong intervals can affect therapeutic blood levels. The use of military time helps to reduce the problem of medications being given at incorrect times.

- The right approach: This involves how one addresses the child and the task at hand, and considers the emotional status and developmental level of the child.

2. Key elements for protocol for administration of medication in a nonmedical setting include the following:

- The child's first and last names are on the container.
- Medication is prescribed by a licensed health professional, and the name, address, and phone number of the health professional who ordered the medication appear on the container.
- Medication is in the original package or container.
- The date the prescription was filled and the date it expires appear on the container.
- Medication is in a childproof container.
- A statement from the healthcare provider indicates the name of the drug, the diagnosis or reason the medication is needed, and whether any serious reactions might occur, or an alert for the nurse about the possibility of a serious drug reaction.
- A policy about self-administration of medication (i.e., the use of inhalers or an EpiPen) should be identified for children who are capable of self-administration, exhibit responsible behaviors, and are in need of speedy access to their medication.
- Information about security and proper storage of medications should be identified in the agency's protocol.
- Nonmedical agencies generally require a written request from the child's parent or guardian asking them to administer the medication per the healthcare provider's specific instruction.

SECTION II: APPLYING YOUR KNOWLEDGE

Activity F **CONSIDER THE SCENARIO AND ANSWER THE QUESTIONS.**

1. 34.1 kg
2. 250 mg
3. 6.25 mL

$$\frac{250 \text{ mg}}{x} = \frac{200 \text{ mg}}{5 \text{ mL}}$$

Cross multiply: $1{,}250 = 200x$. Solve for x: $1{,}250/200 = 6.25$ mL

4. Yes, this is a safe dose.

Low range: 34.1 kg × 0.5 mg = 17 mg/day
High range: 34.1 kg × 2mg = 68.2 mg/day
15 mg × 2 (doses per day) = 30 mg/day

5. a. 340-mg/dose of Tylenol
   b. Dose that should be given is one 325-mg tablet.

10 mg × 34.1kg = 340 mg

SECTION III: PRACTICING FOR NCLEX

Activity G **ANSWER THE FOLLOWING QUESTIONS.**

1. **Answer: c**
   RATIONALE: Most medications are excreted in breast milk. *Medications and Mother's Milk* is an excellent reference to use when determining what medications are suitable for a nursing mother to take. The pediatrician should be notified of the mother's medications. Judgmental statements are inappropriate in the clinical setting and it is not necessary to have breast milk analyzed.

2. **Answer: c**
   RATIONALE: The practitioner who prescribed the medication in question should always be called to verify a proper dose. Asking the previous nurse what she gave or asking the mother if this dose is normal for her son is inappropriate. A medication dose that falls out of the safe range should never be given without verifying the accuracy of the order with the prescribing practitioner.

3. **Answer: d**
   RATIONALE: An oral dose of medication may be readministered if it was vomited less than 5 minutes after it was given. Medication should never be cut in half nor should the frequency be changed.

4. **Answer: a**
   RATIONALE: If a medication error is made, notify the prescriber and pharmacist immediately. Apologizing to the patient is not recommended. Follow your policy with regard to proper documentation of the medication error.

5. **Answer: b**
   RATIONALE: Soliciting the aid of the parents can be especially useful, because they may have already developed a method of medication administration that is acceptable to the child. Using medicine as a treat or reward is not recommended. Do not deceive the child about the fact that you are administering medication.

6. **Answer: a**
   RATIONALE: Squirting a small amount of medicine via a syringe into the infant's cheek is the preferred administration. Never mix medication with the infant's formula or necessary food source (e.g., cereal) or with the child's favorite food. Older children may plug their nose to lessen the taste. Infant's are unable to drink medicine from a medicine cup.

7. **Answer: b**
   RATIONALE: A child must have been walking for at least a year before the dorsogluteal site is used. Even then, the muscle is small, poorly developed, and close to the sciatic nerve, which is relatively large in young children. Therefore, the ventrogluteal or vastus lateralis site is a safer choice in an infant. It is all right for a child to make noise or

cry out during the injection. Also, a 25G needle is used for neonates, not a 1-year-old.

8. **Answer: c**
   RATIONALE: Instructing the child to pant like a puppy provides distraction and relaxes the anal sphincter. Positioning the child in a left lateral position, with the right leg flexed or in the knee–chest position, exposes the anus and helps relax the external sphincter for ease of insertion. Lubricate the suppository with a water-soluble lubricating jelly; petrolatum is an oil-based jelly. If the suppository must be cut to obtain the ordered dose, then it must be cut lengthwise, not crosswise.

9. **Answer: c**
   RATIONALE: Have the child lie in a supine position with his or her head turned to the appropriate side. Pull the earlobe down and back for children younger than 3 years of age. Pulling the ear up and back is appropriate for children older than 3 years of age. Cold medication may cause discomfort and produce vomiting or vertigo in the child. Be careful not to touch the dropper to the ear to prevent contamination of the dropper with microorganisms.

10. **Answer: b**
    RATIONALE: The proper position for the child is in the supine position, with the nurse placing her dominant hand on the child's forehead, and gently pulling back the lower lid to expose the conjunctival sac and placing medication in the inner canthus of the sac. Always clean from the inner canthus to the outer canthus. Medication should not be placed directly onto the cornea. Have the child keep his or her eyes closed for only 1 minute, not 5 minutes.

11. **Answer: a**
    RATIONALE: For a 6-year-old, it is appropriate to offer a choice of what to drink when taking oral medication. Medication should never be compared with candy. Using abstract explanations is appropriate for the adolescent patient only. A child should never be given the opportunity to refuse a medication.

12. **Answer: d**
    RATIONALE: It is acceptable to place a 6-month-old child in your lap to stabilize them as you slowly give the medication by syringe in the side of the mouth. Asking parents to leave is never a good approach; they are a valuable resource for help. This child is much too young to understand a simple explanation.

13. **Answer: c**
    RATIONALE: To obtain the correct dose, you must first convert 28 lb into kg (28/2.2 = 12.7kg). Next you must multiply the number of kilograms by the dose of 5 mg/kg (12.7 × 5 = 63.5 mg). Last, you

must determine how many millimeters to administer using the equation

$$\frac{63.5 \text{ mg}}{x} = \frac{100 \text{ mg}}{5 \text{ mL}}$$

Cross multiply: 317.5 = 100x. Solve for x: 317.5/100 = 3.18 mL

14. **Answer: b**
    RATIONALE: Verbal orders for medication should only be taken during an emergency situation. Requesting the physician to write the order in the chart and explaining the policy is the best response. Refusing to write the order and questioning the medication choice in front of a 14-year-old patient is inappropriate.

15. **Answer: a**
    RATIONALE: The prescribing person should be notified when a child has thrown up the same medication twice. It is not appropriate to put off calling the doctor or put off the mother's concerns for a later time.

CHAPTER 10

SECTION I: ASSESSING YOUR UNDERSTANDING

Activity A FILL IN THE BLANKS.

1. Nociception
2. Dysesthesia
3. Hyperalgesia
4. Allodynia
5. Crying
6. Multimodal
7. Oral
8. Tolerance
9. Iontophoresis
10. Chronic
11. Fifth vital sign

Activity B MATCH THE TYPES OF ANALGESIA MEDICATION ADMINISTRATION IN COLUMN A WITH THEIR DISADVANTAGES IN COLUMN B.

| 1. j | 2. h | 3. d | 4. g | 5. b |
| 6. i | 7. e | 8. a | 9. f | 10. c |

Activity C WRITE THE CORRECT SEQUENCE OF NOCICEPTION IN THE BOXES PROVIDED.

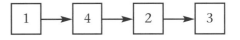

Activity D BRIEFLY ANSWER THE FOLLOWING.

1. The three types of pain relief medications used with children are nonopioids, opioids, and co-analgesics.

   a. Nonopioid Analgesics: Nonopioid analgesics are indicated for mild to moderate pain or for use in conjunction with opioids for moderate to severe pain to augment and decrease opioid requirements. They work well for musculoskeletal pain. Nonopioids differ from opioids in that they are antipyretic, have a ceiling effect, and do not produce tolerance or physical or psychological dependence. Nonopioid analgesics include acetaminophen and nonsteroidal anti-inflammatory drugs, such as ibuprofen.

   b. Opioid Analgesics: Opioid analgesics are indicated for moderate to severe pain that is not relieved with nonopioids. Opioids differ from nonopioids in that they do not have an antipyretic effect or a ceiling of analgesia. Therefore, opioids will not mask fever, and opioid doses can be titrated upward until pain is relieved or intolerable side effects develop. Physical dependence on opioids develops in as little as 7 days of continuous use.

   c. Co-analgesics: Co-analgesics include medications such as tricyclic antidepressants, selective serotonin reuptake inhibitors (SSRIs), anticonvulsants, benzodiazepines, and local anesthetics. These drugs play a role in pain management by potentiating the effects of analgesics, treating the side effects of analgesics, or exerting an analgesic effect of their own.

2. The following are the four stages of Nociception:

   a. Transduction: Tissue injury from trauma, surgery, or disease releases chemical mediators such as prostaglandins, bradykinin, serotonin, norepinephrine, substance P, and histamine, which cause pain at the periphery and facilitate movement of pain impulses along peripheral nerves. Primary afferent fibers, most commonly A delta and C fibers, when excited by mechanical, thermal, or chemical stimuli, depolarize and transmit information about noxious stimuli from the periphery to the dorsal horn of the spinal cord.

   b. Transmission: All incoming information related to pain crosses the dorsal horn of the spinal cord on its entry into the central nervous system (CNS). Neurotransmitters (adenosine triphosphate, glutamate, substance P) continue the pain impulse from the peripheral nociceptors to the dorsal horn neurons. The signals are transmitted through the CNS to the brain stem, thalamus, and the cerebral cortex.

   c. Perception: At this level of nociception, the person becomes conscious of the pain. Several central structures are involved in pain perception; no single "pain center" exists. The reticular system is believed to warn the individual to recognize pain and initiate an autonomic response. The somatosensory cortex provides recognition of the location and quality of the pain. The limbic system initiates the emotional and behavioral response to pain. Cognitive and behavioral techniques, such as distraction and guided imagery, modify pain perception by directing the cortical structures to attend to competing information.

   d. Modulation: The CNS rapidly sends descending messages back through the dorsal horn, thus inhibiting the transmission of noxious stimuli. Neurotransmitters such as endorphins, enkephalins, serotonin, norepinephrine, GABA, and neurotensin modulate pain. Baclofen and antidepressants (e.g., the tricyclics and some SSRIs) are used to modulate chronic pain at this level of nociception.

SECTION II: APPLYING YOUR KNOWLEDGE

Activity E CONSIDER THE SCENARIO AND ANSWER THE QUESTIONS.

1. Aiden is 9 years old and capable of describing his pain on a numeric scale. The parents should be taught how to assess Aiden's pain using a numeric scale, such as a 0- to 10-poin scale with 0 point representing no pain and 10 points representing excruciating or unbearable pain. The parents could also be taught to determine pain level by observing physical symptoms such as guarding, facial grimace, teeth clenching, and so forth.

2. Aiden's parents should be given a list of medications that he is to given for pain postoperatively. This should include medication name, strength, dosing interval, and route to be given. Aiden's parents should also be given a plan for treating mild, moderate, and severe pain.

SECTION III: PRACTICING FOR NCLEX

Activity F ANSWER THE FOLLOWING QUESTIONS.

1. **Answer: c**
   RATIONALE: Developmentally appropriate pain intensity scales can be used to obtain a self-report from children as young as 3 years of age (Zempsky & Schechter, 2003).

2. **Answer: a**
   RATIONALE: By 4 years of age, children have learned to control their facial expressions and may mask facial indications of pain (Gaffney et al., 2003).

3. **Answer: b**
   RATIONALE: Gaze aversion, hiccups, yawning, and flaccid posture are all physical indicators of stress in a preterm infant. The remaining indicators include indicators of pain in other developmental stages.

4. **Answer: d**
   RATIONALE: Parents who are knowledgeable about what is going to happen and about specific things they can do to facilitate pain management generally feel less helpless, are less anxious, and are better able to support their children. A parent's sensitive response to a child's reaction can promote the child's coping skills during a painful procedure.

5. **Answer: c**
   RATIONALE: The distraction must be unique and powerful enough to hold the child's attention; therefore, fewer attentional resources are available to focus on distressing and painful stimuli. The distraction must be age appropriate. Action video games have demonstrated a unique ability to engross teenagers' attention. The other distracters are not developmentally appropriate for James.

6. **Answer: a**
   RATIONALE: Deep breathing is a common relaxation intervention. This activity can help relax tense muscles before the injection. Loud music can further excite the child. Turning off the lights may frighten a child. Just telling a child to relax serves no purpose. Also, the child may have no experience at a beach to draw from.

7. **Answer: c**
   RATIONALE: Swaddling and holding is comforting, and helps infants and small children achieve a more relaxed state. Facilitated tucking (in which the caregiver places a hand on the infant's head and feet while providing flexion and containment), swaddling, and other positional interventions serve to limit excessive, uncontrolled movements that may exacerbate pain. Holding down the newborn's arms and legs as well as holding them away from the body can be further stressful to the newborn.

8. **Answer: d**
   RATIONALE: Ice massage is effective for injection pain, headaches, toothaches, or brief, painful procedures. Ice or cold packs should not be used for more than 15 minutes. Heat is most effective in relieving pain from inflammation and spasm. Gentle muscle massage is helpful; however, the most effective pain relief method is the ice massage.

9. **Answer: b**
   RATIONALE: Continuously monitor the child's oxygen saturation and heart rate, and also document vital signs such as heart rate, respiratory rate, blood pressure, oxygen saturation, and level of consciousness at least every 5 minutes during sedation of a child.

10. **Answer: b**
    RATIONALE: Before administering opioid medications in the emergency department, assessment for shock and head injury must be completed first. Parental permission is not necessary. Opioid medications are appropriate for severe pain after assessments for head injury and shock have been completed.

11. **Answer: a**
    RATIONALE: Aspirin may be used to manage chronic inflammatory disease such as juvenile rheumatoid arthritis.

12. **Answer: c**
    RATIONALE: The Faces pain scale is recommended for children as young as 3 years of age. The visual analogue scale and the numeric rating scale are for children age 7 years and older. A child must be able to read and write to use the pain diary.

13. **Answer: c**
    RATIONALE: The FLACC scale can be used with infants and also with children who are nonverbal. The Faces scale and the numeric rating scale require verbal interaction with the patient and would not be appropriate for this nonverbal patient. The Varni-Thompson Pediatric Pain Questionnaire is recommended for children 8 years and older and also requires verbal communication.

14. **Answer: c**
    RATIONALE: Baclofen or antidepressants are analgesics of choice when controlling pain at the modulation stage of nociception. Nonopioids are useful during the transduction stage and opioids are useful during the transmission stage.

Activity G **CHOOSE ALL ANSWERS THAT APPLY.**

1. **Answer: a, b, c, d**
   RATIONALE: Disrupted sleep patterns, normal vital signs, depression, and developmental regression would all be common findings of a child who experiences chronic pain.

2. **Answer: a, c**
   RATIONALE: The preschool-aged child fears bodily injury and mutilation, and also needs some control of the situation. The preschool child has words to describe pain and does not have the ability to delay gratification.

3. **Answer: b, c**
   RATIONALE: The preterm infant has a shorter, higher pitched cry, which arouses the listener; the posture of a preterm infant can be listless, limp, or flaccid. A toddler will have a facial grimace, clenched teeth, tightly shut lips or biting lips, wide open eyes, and a wrinkled forehead. Preterm infants are unable to withdraw a limb.

4. **Answer: a, b, c, d**
   RATIONALE: The indicators that a child is suitable for PCA medication include that the child is able to quantify pain, the child is unable to tolerate oral analgesics, the child understands the relation between pushing the button and receiving medication, and the child reports unsatisfactory pain relief with the current regimen.

5. **Answer: a, b, d**
   RATIONALE: Urinary retention, constipation, nausea and vomiting, sedation, pruritus, and respiratory depression are all common side effect of opioids.

CHAPTER 11

SECTION I: ASSESSING YOUR UNDERSTANDING

Activity A FILL IN THE BLANKS.

1. Acute illness
2. Atraumatic
3. Immobilization
4. Standard precautions
5. Playroom
6. Animal-assisted therapy
7. Elbow immobilizers
8. Mummy immobilization
9. Consent form
10. Bronchospasm

Activity B MATCH THE TYPES OF ATRAUMATIC CARE NURSING INTERVENTIONS IN COLUMN A WITH THE ASPECT OF CARE THEY FOCUS ON IN COLUMN B.

1. d   2. e   3. f   4. b   5. h
6. i   7. a   8. c   9. g

Activity C WRITE THE CORRECT SEQUENCE OF PATIENT EDUCATION IN THE BOXES PROVIDED.

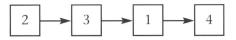

Activity D BRIEFLY ANSWER THE FOLLOWING.

1. The three stages of separation anxiety are as follows:

   - Protest: During this phase, which lasts hours to days, the child searches for the lost parent, angrily protests, cries frequently, and rejects hospital staff. When the parent returns, the child readily goes to him or her.
   - Despair: During this phase, the child becomes more sad and apathetic, mourning the lost parent; however, he or she cries less and searches the environment less. The child makes few demands on the environment and those within it. When the parent returns, the child may not readily approach him or her, or may cling to the parent.
   - Denial: During this phase, the child becomes cheerful, interested in the environment and new persons, and seemingly unaware of the lost parent. The child is friendly with staff and begins to develop superficial relationships. When the parent returns, the child typically ignores them as a coping mechanism to avoid further emotional pain. Children who progress to denial, however, suffer long-term impaired parental relationships and impaired trust, which can lead to problems in establishing close relationships, attention deficits, self-centeredness, and decreased intellectual functioning.

2. If parents are absent as a result of work, sibling care, or other responsibilities, reinforce that the child will be attended to in their absence. Provide the family with the name and telephone number of a contact person knowledgeable about the child; the nurse can also initiate regular telephone contact with the family. When appropriate, assist the child in calling home.

3. The advantages of care conferences include the following:

   - Promote clear, effective communication between the family and members of the healthcare team.
   - Facilitate collaboration between the family and healthcare team.
   - Facilitate the identification of priorities and development of a comprehensive plan of care to address psychosocial, physical, and developmental needs of the hospitalized child and family.
   - Ensure adequate preparation for discharge and transition to home.

SECTION II: APPLYING YOUR KNOWLEDGE

Activity E CONSIDER THE SCENARIO AND ANSWER THE QUESTIONS.

1. Address the parents' anxiety and assess the cause. Reassure the parents with complete explanations of what to expect and answer all questions. The parents' anxiety level has a direct effect on the child, so you will want to decrease their anxiety level as much as you are able.

2. Give the child a simple explanation of the procedure in concrete terms before beginning. Prior to the IV insertion, use a topical anesthetic on two locations suitable for an IV. Allow time for the anesthetic time to become effective. Attempt to place the IV in a location where the child or infant will not need a lot of restraints or arm boards. If not possible, use padded or air-filled arm boards of the appropriate size, with a nonthreatening look (e.g., colorful covers with pediatric designs) to provide extra cushioning.

3. Discharge teaching after surgery would include pain medication doses and administration, signs and symptoms of postoperative infection, typical postanesthesia behaviors (lethargy, decreased appetite, crankiness), incision care, activity limitations, and follow-up appointments.

SECTION III: PRACTICING FOR NCLEX

Activity F CHOOSE ALL ANSWERS THAT APPLY.

1. **Answer: b**
   RATIONALE: Family-centered care encourages liberal 24-hour visitation policies, sibling involvement in hospitalization, pet visitation policies, family conferences to promote shared decision making, assisting families to utilize support systems, and family education with regard to the care of the child. A weekly patient care conference doesn't necessarily mean the parents will be included in the meeting. An expectation that parents are continually present to provide all care can increase parent stress. Assess the parents' desire for involvement and explicitly negotiate boundaries of care.

2. **Answer: c**
   RATIONALE: Frequency and timing of bathing are often culturally determined. Respect habits within the confines of standards acceptable for infection control and scheduling. Some children are accustomed to bathing in the morning, whereas others prefer to bathe before bed. Keep as close to the home routine as possible to decrease stress while in the hospital. Daily baths are not necessary. Discouraging parent involvement in the infant's bath does not promote family-centered care. Instruct the parents how to bathe the infant without dislodging the IV. A 6-month-old will not be able to stand unassisted. A better assessment would be to determine whether the infant can sit in a tub unassisted.

3. **Answer: c**
   RATIONALE: Allowing the hospitalized child to use a familiar toothbrush from home may encourage good oral hygiene. Although it is important to permit preschool-aged children to begin brushing their own teeth, they need one thorough brushing per day with the assistance of an adult. Washing the gums with a cloth or sponge is appropriate for infants. A fluoride rinse may be used with older children who are able to rinse and spit.

4. **Answer: b**
   RATIONALE: Encourage the child to choose the clothes they wear. This may be especially important to adolescents, whose chief developmental concerns are body image and personal appearance. Forcing a child to wear a gown limits their control and adds stress. Hospital gowns are not necessarily cleaner than clothes from home.

5. **Answer: d**
   RATIONALE: Being direct and matter-of-fact, and allowing as much privacy as possible are the preferred interventions in these situations. Keeping toileting implements, such as urinals and bedpans, out of sight when not in use and keeping bedside

commodes emptied, clean, and stored as covertly as possible are also commonsense interventions related to toileting. Promptly answering the call light promotes trust that assistance is available when needed. This decreases a sense of humiliation and anxiety.

6. **Answer: a**
   RATIONALE: To reduce risk of SIDS, place infants supine for sleep and do not use soft objects or soft bedding in the crib for infants or for the child who is developmentally delayed until the child can lift and turn his or her head.

7. **Answer: c**
   RATIONALE: Assessment of home preferences and routines for sleeping are steps toward eliminating sleep pattern disturbance in the hospital. Determining the child's bedtime, sleep duration, bedtime rituals, and nap pattern helps the nurse develop a plan of care that prevents sleep pattern disturbance.

8. **Answer: b**
   RATIONALE: The proper identification procedure involves verifying the child's identity with two identifiers (e.g., name, date of birth, medical record number), and matching the service about to be performed (by checking the medication label, laboratory requisition, medical record). It is not permissible to use a bed number or only verbally verify the child's name.

9. **Answer: b**
   RATIONALE: Exhaust all alternatives to immobilization (e.g., distraction, parental or staff presence) before using any restraint, and implement the least restrictive methods first. Never use a restraint to discipline a child, to place them in a time-out. Never tie immobilizers to bedside rails, because raising or lowering of the rail could injure the immobilized limb.

10. **Answer: c**
    RATIONALE: It is unsafe to carry a child for a long distance because of the risk of tripping, slipping, falling, or fatiguing. Walking for a distance is not an appropriate option for sick children. Use transport devices, such as wheelchairs and stretchers, to transport children from the pediatric unit to other areas of the hospital, such as radiology or the laboratory. Also, never leave a pediatric patient alone when being transported.

11. **Answer: a**
    RATIONALE: The best treatment for latex allergy is identification of high-risk populations and minimizing latex exposure in these children. Using nonlatex gloves, using nonlatex IV tubing, and drawing up medications in syringes just prior to use are good ways to decrease exposure; however, identification of the high-risk patient is the first priority.

12. Answer: a, b, c, d

RATIONALE: Most of the missing children in the United States are abducted by one of their own parents. Some of these abductions occur when the family is experiencing unusual circumstances, such as hospitalization for an acute illness. Proper patient and visitor identification policies along with a well-planned and structured infant and child security program within the hospital setting can prevent child abductions and provide a safe environment for the acutely ill child.

13. Answer: c

RATIONALE: The adolescent suffers separation anxiety when separated from peers rather than parents. Separation anxiety can be experienced by children of all ages. Separation anxiety is not resolved as soon as the parent returns. This anxiety can be described in three stages. Children who progress to the final stage, denial, can suffer long-term impaired parental relationships and impaired trust, which can lead to problems in establishing close relationships, attention deficits, self-centeredness, and decreased intellectual functioning.

14. Answer: a, b, c

RATIONALE: The use of play, drawing pictures, and listening to music can all be appropriate tools to help children cope with the stresses of the acute care setting. Encouraging destructive behavior is not an acceptable method of coping.

15. Answer: a

RATIONALE: Family-centered care also addresses the needs of siblings. Encourage parents to have the sibling visit and be included in the plan of care. Sibling visitation can clear up misconceptions and feelings of jealousy that the sibling might have.

16. Answer: a, c, d

RATIONALE: Preoperative anxiety has been identified as a universal phenomenon and can be expected to affect young children as well as older patients. Children's anxiety is related to their parents' anxiety. Use videos, tours, pictures, manipulation of medical equipment, or role playing to increase the effectiveness of the information, and help allay fears and correct misconceptions.

17. Answer: c

RATIONALE: The parent or legal guardian is asked to sign a consent form when a child is admitted to the hospital. In an emergency, when a delay in obtaining consent is likely to lead to loss of the patient's life or significant functioning, the physician can authorize an emergency procedure.

18. Answer: b

RATIONALE: Children with neuromuscular disorders may be at risk for increased intracranial pressure as a result of cerebral vasodilation during induction. Premature infants are at increased risk for developing postoperative apnea during the first 6 months of life. Children with asthma are at risk for bronchospasm, and children in general are at risk for anesthesia-related cardiac arrest.

19. Answer: a, b, c, d

RATIONALE: Preventing the negative effects that long-term hospitalizations can have involves maintaining consistent caregivers, early developmental intervention, and taking infants to the playroom and obtaining schooling for older children.

20. Answer: d

RATIONALE: Have the parents assume total care of the child in the hospital for 24 hours to gain familiarity and comfort with the process while still having medical support close by. Making a follow-up appointment, completing discharge paperwork, and completing a satisfaction survey is helpful, but the having the parents care for the child is the best intervention.

CHAPTER 12

SECTION I: ASSESSING YOUR UNDERSTANDING

Activity A MATCH THE TERMS IN COLUMN A WITH THE DESCRIPTION OR RELATED STATEMENT FROM COLUMN B.

1. a   **2.** d   **3.** e   **4.** b   **5.** c

Activity B FILL IN THE BLANKS.

1. Multiple
2. Exacerbation
3. Complication
4. Preschool
5. Younger

Activity C SUPPLY THE INFORMATION REQUESTED.

1. a. Avoid
   b. Avoid
   c. Appropriate
   d. Appropriate
   e. Avoid
   f. Avoid
   g. Appropriate
   h. Avoid
   i. Avoid
2. The ADA definition of disability focuses on key life functions that are expected of a child of a particular age. The IDEA definition of disability is characterized by disorders that will qualify a student for special education and related services.
3. Chronic illness implies being sick and needing to recover. For example, cancer is a chronic illness for which the goal is remission of symptoms; often, the healthcare community begins to use the term

cured after five years or more without symptoms. On the other hand, the vast majority of chronic conditions are not chronic illnesses. A chronic condition, such as Down syndrome or asthma, is always present and, although the individual may also become ill during a period of exacerbation, their chronic condition is not a illness from which they can recover.

SECTION II: APPLYING YOUR KNOWLEDGE

Activity D CONSIDER THE SCENARIO AND ANSWER THE QUESTIONS.

1. It is important for the nurse to understand that each family responds to a chronic condition differently. The nurse's role is to understand and assist families dealing with a child with a chronic condition. The nurse assists families through specific times when the stress of the condition is greater, assists potential stressors, provides support, and facilitates coping. In Melissa's case, the increasing symptoms have caused increased stress on the family. The nurse should assess the family support, family dynamics, and provide appropriate resources to help the family through the adjustment period. Teaching of the new medicine regime would be important, as well as assessing the affect of Melissa's absenteeism on her school. The nurse needs to provide guidance and reassurance to Melissa that she should continue to play tennis and participate in activities as usual unless she in not feeling well.

2. The nurse would act as an advocate for Melissa and her family in managing the condition, with teaching as an ongoing process, because knowledge of the condition and treatment helps to decrease stress. The nurse also teaches the parents and the child the necessary skills to care for the condition. Further education will be needed as the condition changes. In addition, the nurse would assist the family to develop a care routine; identify, assess, and coordinate community resources; and assess ongoing coping mechanisms.

   In Melissa's case the goal as is to promote as much normalcy as possible. Possible referrals to community resources such as a nutritionist, psychologist, and social services may be helpful. Frequent and open communication with the school and school nurse will be important in facilitating Melissa's success in school and not falling behind with frequent absences. Also, a tutor may be helpful to assist her to keep up with homework during periods of exacerbations. Referral to a camp or support group so that Melissa can meet other teenagers with the same or other chronic conditions provides more normalcy. Mary should be referred to social services to obtain information on potential finan-

cial assistance and planning for the future, helping her through the insurance maze to access the services the child needs without depriving the family of its needs.

SECTION III: PRACTICING FOR NCLEX

Activity E CHOOSE THE ANSWER THAT IS THE BEST ANSWER FOR EACH QUESTION.

1. a   **2.** c   **3.** b   **4.** a   **5.** d
6. d

CHAPTER 13

SECTION I: ASSESSING YOUR UNDERSTANDING

Activity A FILL IN THE BLANKS.

1. 1. 7% to 10%
2. Palliative care
3. Hospice
4. Meperidine (Demerol)
5. 4 to 6 months
6. Respite care
7. Grief
8. Bereavement
9. Siblings
10. Parent

Activity B MATCH THE TYPES OF GRIEF IN COLUMN A WITH THEIR DEFINITION IN COLUMN B.

1. d   **2.** c   **3.** e   **4.** a   **5.** f
6. b

Activity C WRITE THE CORRECT SEQUENCE OF THE FIVE STAGES OF GRIEF ACCORDING TO KUBLER-ROSS.

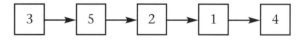

Activity D BRIEFLY ANSWER THE FOLLOWING.

1. The need for palliative care exists for children with the following conditions:
   - Life-threatening conditions for which treatment is available but may fail
   - Cancer
   - Conditions in which premature death is expected, but long periods of intensive treatment

to prolong good quality of life are anticipated (cystic fibrosis, HIV)

- Progressive conditions that may extend over many years and for which no curative treatment is available (mucopolysaccharidosis).
- Conditions with severe disability that, although not progressive, lead to extreme vulnerability and in which premature death is likely (cerebral palsy)
- Neonatal conditions in which the diagnosis of a terminal condition may be made prenatally or is evident at birth

2. The Last Acts five core principles from which palliative care must be integrated throughout the trajectory of a child's illness are as follows:

- Respecting patient goals, preferences, and choices
- Providing comprehensive care
- Using the strength of interdisciplinary resources
- Acknowledging and addressing caregiver concerns
- Building systems that support responsible palliative care policies and regulations

3. The Initiative for Pediatric Palliative Care's (IPPC) four cornerstones of clinical practice in pediatric palliative care are as follows:

- Responding to the ethical claim of the child/family
- Adopting a collaborative relational stance
- Cultivating cultural humility
- Developing reflective practice

SECTION II: APPLYING YOUR KNOWLEDGE
Activity E CONSIDER THE SCENARIO AND ANSWER THE QUESTIONS.

1. Tell the parents they may take their son home after arrangements for care at home have been made.
2. Since John has only 2 months left, the best resource would be hospice care if they plan to take him home to die.
3. Tell the parents to be truthful when discussing John's condition. Jack can be given information in simple and concrete terms. Samantha will need more explanation than her brother. Advise the Schneiders to involve the siblings in the care at home and the decisions made involving end-of-life activities such as funeral planning. Encourage them not to involve themselves so completely in John's death that they forget the needs of their other children.

SECTION III: PRACTICING FOR NCLEX
Activity F CHOOSE ALL ANSWERS THAT APPLY.

1. **Answer: b**
   RATIONALE: Cultivating cultural humility, the third premise, expresses the need to reflect on one's

own culture as well as the culture of the child and the family. This requires the capacity for awareness and self-critique regarding one's own culture and beliefs. Answers a, c, and d describe the other three cornerstones.

2. **Answer: d**
   RATIONALE: Nurses can help the family by establishing a relationship, by being present both physically and emotionally, and by continuing to focus on the family as a system. Individual focus at this time is not appropriate. Focus also on adding life to the years, not years to the life, of the child.

3. **Answer: b**
   RATIONALE: There is often disparity between the way children die and the way they want to be cared for when dying. Most healthcare workers report a lack of education on death and dying. Families often have a difficult time accepting the reality of the dying child.

4. **Answer: d**
   RATIONALE: According to Children's Hospice International (CHI), fewer than 1% of children in the United States who could benefit from hospice services receive it.

5. **Answer: c**
   RATIONALE: It is not until children reach school age that they understand that death is permanent and irreversible.

6. **Answer: d**
   RATIONALE: Terminal dehydration and anorexia do not cause suffering in the individual who has no desire for food and water. When a child has reached the stage of terminal dehydration and anorexia, it is not appropriate to initiate enteral or parenteral feedings, because they do not promote comfort at this point and will not sustain life. Education to families is crucial to help them understand that these are common and natural components of the dying process.

7. **Answer: c**
   RATIONALE: School plays a very important part in a child's life. In addition to helping the child acquire knowledge, school activities promote self-esteem and allow the child to be identified as an important member of society. At school, the child can continue to gain independence and maintain some degree of control over the environment. This should be discussed with the parents and the doctor to see if this is viable.

8. **Answer: c**
   RATIONALE: Daily weights and lab work are futile and often omitted from care. Withholding parenteral or enteral nutrition in a child who is hungry in not appropriate. Suctioning and oxygen can provide comfort and therefore should not be omitted. Likewise, antibiotics should not be omitted because urinary tract infections can cause pain to the dying child.

9. **Answer: a**

   RATIONALE: In cases of severe injuries, prepare the parents for how the child looks. Prepare the child and room for the parents' visit, but it might be beneficial to leave much of the resuscitation equipment in the room to reinforce the fact that efforts were taken to save the child. Parents who do not want to see their child after the death can be gently encouraged to do so. Even when the death was the result of severe trauma, parents who see their child have fewer fantasies about the event.

10. **Answer: b**

    RATIONALE: When a child is at the funeral of a family member, advise parents to have a person sit with the siblings to answer questions or take them out if they feel they need to leave during the service. Regardless of the child's cultural background, allow siblings of a child who has died to be involved to the degree that they wish to be involved. Siblings do not need to be protected from the death process.

11. **Answer: c**

    RATIONALE: Care should be taken to bathe the infant, then dress and swaddle in a blanket before presenting the infant to the mother. Be cautious about allowing fathers or other family members to decide whether the mother is to see her deceased child. Offer this opportunity to the infant's mother independent of family input. Comments such as reminding a mother of her healthy children at home diminish the loss of that specific pregnancy.

12. **Answer: a, b, c, d**

    RATIONALE: Recognizing the loss; reacting to the separation; recollecting and reexperiencing the deceased and the relationship; relinquishing old attachments to the deceased and to the shared world; readjusting to allow movement into a new world without the loved one, but without forgetting the old world; and reinvesting in the new world are all bereavement tasks.

13. **Answer: b, c, d**

    RATIONALE: Don't be afraid that mentioning the child will remind them of their grief. A hug or a hand to hold can sometimes say more than words. Say "I'm sorry." After you have expressed your sorrow, allow the parents or family to respond. Don't be afraid of silence. Often, your caring presence is enough. There are many helpful things to do, but shielding the family from the reality of the situation is not one of them.

14. **Answer: a, b, c**

    RATIONALE: Elevating the head of the bed can ease the work of breathing. Offering reassurance to the family that agonal breaths are a normal part of dying is helpful. Offering a quiet and calm environment is also helpful because agonal breaths can be very stressful for the family. Massage is not helpful at this time.

15. **Answer: a, b, c, d**

    RATIONALE: All of these interventions would be suitable for the sibling of a child who has died. Sharing feelings help children to vent their emotions and work through their grief. Touch can be very comforting after the loss of a loved one. Sharing your memories helps the sibling feel your affection for the child. Involving the sibling helps that child feel a part of the process.

CHAPTER 14

SECTION I: ASSESSING YOUR UNDERSTANDING

Activity A MATCH THE TERM IN COLUMN A WITH THE DESCRIPTION IN COLUMN B.

1. e   **2.** c   **3.** b   **4.** d   **5.** a

Activity B INDICATE WHETHER THE FOLLOWING STATEMENTS ARE TRUE OR FALSE.

1. T   **2.** F   **3.** T   **4.** F   **5.** F

Activity C FILL IN THE BLANKS.

1. Insulin
2. Sclera
3. Hypoxemia
4. Phenotype

SECTION II: APPLYING YOUR KNOWLEDGE

Activity D CONSIDER THE SCENARIO AND ANSWER THE QUESTIONS.

1. Regina is most likely experiencing hypothermia. Premature infants are at risk for hypothermia. Hypothermic newborns may appear pale, with acrocyanosis or central cyanosis, mottling, and signs of respiratory distress. Chronic hypothermia in newborns may present poor weight gain, metabolic acidosis, apnea, and bradycardia.

   Regina is at risk for hypothermia because the limited ability to produce heat, coupled with many mechanisms of heat loss, make the premature newborn very susceptible to hypothermia. The term newborn is able to increase muscle activity, initiate nonshivering or chemical thermogenesis, and utilize brown fat stores to generate heat. The preterm newborn is unable to increase muscle activity or to assume a flexed position because of poor motor tone, and has limited brown fat stores as well. In addition, premature newborns may be unable to initiate thermogenesis because of limited stores of fat and insufficient amounts of chemicals such as glucose, liver enzymes, and hormones.

2. Preventing cold stress, promoting a neutral thermal environment, and monitoring for hypothermia are cornerstones to caring for all newborns, especially premature infants. Warming scales, stethoscopes, and blankets are other effective interventions to prevent heat loss. The infant may be placed in a double-walled isolette or radiant warmer if his or her temperature is critically low. Initially, the child should be wrapped in warm blankets and placed in an area of the room that is not drafty or near an air vent. Finally, place a cap on the newborn's head, which is an easy and effective intervention to prevent heat loss in the premature newborn. Closely monitor the newborn's skin and core temperatures, as well as the isolette or ambient temperature. Monitor the newborn's core temperature by the axillary route every hour until it is stable, and then every 2 to 3 hours.

Clustering care (performing many tasks at the same time), if the newborn tolerates this approach, is one method to reduce heat loss and limits fluctuations in temperature. Collaborate with other members of the healthcare team to time procedures and examinations to limit heat losses and provide extended sleep periods.

3. At this time, it would not be appropriate for the nurse to allow Louise to bathe Regina because of the hypothermia and temperature instability. Infants lose heat through evaporation during bathing. It should be explained to the mother that because of the infant's inability to utilize brown fat stores to generate heat, and her low temperature, giving a bath at this time would only provide additional stress that would lower her temperature even more. The infant should be treated for the hypothermia and monitored. After the temperature is stable, the infant can be bathed following appropriate procedures to maintain a neutral thermal environment and prevent heat loss.

SECTION III: PRACTICING FOR NCLEX

Activity E   CHOOSE THE BEST ANSWER FOR EACH QUESTION.

1. c   2. d   3. a   4. d   5. c
6. c, d, f

CHAPTER 15

SECTION I: ASSESSING YOUR UNDERSTANDING

Activity A   FILL IN THE BLANKS.

1. Rheumatic heart disease
2. Kawasaki disease
3. Antibiotics
4. Cardiac catheterization
5. Heart failure

Activity B   MATCH THE FOLLOWING CLINICAL SIGNS IN COLUMN B WITH THE TYPE OF JONES CRITERIA IN COLUMN A. YOU MAY USE THE ANSWERS MORE THAN ONCE.

1. a, b, c   2. d   3. e

Activity C   WRITE THE CORRECT PATHOPHYSIOLOGIC SEQUENCING FOR A CHILD IN HEART FAILURE WITH LEFT VENTRICULAR HEART DYSFUNCTION.

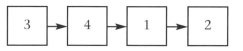

| 3 | → | 4 | → | 1 | → | 2 |

Activity D   BRIEFLY ANSWER THE FOLLOWING.

1. Potential environmental factors that may cause congenital heart defects include the ingestion of drugs or alcohol during pregnancy, and lithium carbonate or aspirin products.
2. Palpate the chest for the apical impulse for placement, and heaves and thrills.
3. The balloon is inflated over the stenotic area and increases the luminal diameter. This improves blood flow through the stenotic area.
4. Provide calming and comforting measures. Oxygen is administered, as well as morphine sulfate. Place the child in the knee–chest position.
5. Primary hypertension is diagnosed if no cause can be found for the elevated blood pressure. Secondary hypertension is diagnosed if the elevated blood pressure results from other pathologies such as renal disease, heart disease, endocrinopathy, or central nervous system changes.

SECTION II: APPLYING YOUR KNOWLEDGE

Activity E   CONSIDER THE SCENARIO AND ANSWER THE QUESTIONS.

1. The nurse should call 911. The practitioner on site needs to be included immediately in the situation. The infant should receive oxygen until the EMT arrives.
2. The probable cause of the cyanosis is a result of the ductus arteriosis closing and the infant has a congenital heart defect, such as hypoplastic left heart syndrome. The nurse can anticipate the infant being transferred to the closest pediatric care hospital for care. The nurse would anticipate attempting to keep the ductus open with an intravenous infusion of prostaglandin E1 and low-dose dopamine to maintain adequate systemic perfusion. The infant will need surgery to correct the defect if possible.

SECTION III: PRACTICING FOR NCLEX

Activity F   BRIEFLY ANSWER THE QUESTIONS.

1. Umbilical vein
2. Coarctation of the aorta
3. Pulmonary artery
4. Inotropic

Activity G   CHOOSE THE BEST ANSWER.

1. **Answer: b**
   RATIONALE: Echocardiograms are performed to determine whether a child has a cardiac defect. Many heart murmurs are normal and considered innocent, so an echocardiogram is not routine for all murmurs. This test does not measure the impulses of the heart—that is an EKG.

2. **Answer: a**
   RATIONALE: Heart defects are commonly associated with Down syndrome, which is the most likely explanation. Medication and environmental factors may have an effect on the developing heart, but children with Down syndrome often have this association. The echocardiogram will not determine the cause of the heart defect.

3. **Answer: b**
   RATIONALE: Poor feeding would be one of the signs of a cardiac defect in an infant. It would be difficult to assess whether the infant is having chest pain or vertigo. A rash is not a sign of a cardiac defect.

4. **Answer: d**
   RATIONALE: Respiratory rate is part of the cardiovascular assessment. Range of motion, head circumference, and newborn reflexes would be important to assess, but they are not necessarily the most important part of the newborn assessment.

5. **Answer: d**
   RATIONALE: This is an invasive test that can also provide an intervention of the heart if needed. It can check the size of the vessels within the heart. This test does not check the size of the heart, electrical impulses of the heart, or how blood is flowing through the heart.

6. **Answer: a**
   RATIONALE: Having the child meet someone in a cardiac catheterization uniform will help decrease the child's anxiety about the procedure. If the child has a fever, the procedure would be postponed. An IV line would not usually be placed in the foot.

7. **Answer: a**
   RATIONALE: Children with hypoplastic left heart usually need several surgeries. There is not a surgery that will cure the heart defect. The surgery is not exploratory.

8. **Answer: c**
   RATIONALE: A central IV will allow continuous monitoring of blood pressure. The peripheral IV will not monitor blood pressure, and a blood pressure cuff is not a continuous measurement. The probes on the chest wall do not measure blood pressure.

9. **Answer: b**
   RATIONALE: Albumin is an intravascular volume expander. It will not increase fluid volume and it is not a vasodilator.

10. **Answer: a**
    RATIONALE: Poor capillary refill and cold extremities could be a sign of a cardiovascular problem, especially if the child has a cardiac defect. Respiratory distress and a medication allergy are highly unlikely. This is not a normal finding in a child.

CHAPTER 16

SECTION I: ASSESSING YOUR UNDERSTANDING

Activity A   MATCH THE TERM IN COLUMN A WITH THE DESCRIPTION FROM COLUMN B.

1. f	2. h	3. g	4. d	5. c
6. e	7. b	8. a		

Activity B   INDICATE WHETHER THE FOLLOWING STATEMENTS ARE TRUE OR FALSE.

1. F	2. T	3. F	4. T	5. F

Activity C   FILL IN THE BLANKS.

1. Prone
2. Clear
3. Ethmoid, maxillary, sphenoid, frontal
4. School-aged
5. Apnea

SECTION II: APPLYING YOUR KNOWLEDGE

Activity D   CONSIDER THE SCENARIO AND ANSWER THE QUESTIONS.

1. Dominic has a clear, watery nasal discharge with nasal congestion; itchy, watery eyes; no fever; and no sore throat. In addition, his mother reports that he experiences similar symptoms around the same time each year, suggesting a seasonal nature. These would help to support the diagnosis of allergic rhinitis. If Dominic had a cold, he would most likely have a fever, purulent nasal secretions, and pharyngitis or laryngitis.

   The nurse would need to determine whether Dominic has a familial predisposition to allergic rhinitis and whether Dominic has experienced any fatigue, irritability, headache, depression, or anorexia. In addition, the nurse would look for certain characteristic features, such as a bluish discoloration of the infraorbital area (*allergic shiners*), a transverse crease across the lower third of the nose (as a result of rubbing the nose; *allergic salute*), and pale-pink to blue-gray turbinates.

2. Medication therapy involves the use of oral or intranasal antihistamines, decongestants, intranasal corticosteroids, leukotriene modifiers, mast cell stabilizers, and allergen-specific immunotherapy. Antihistamines are used to block histamine from binding at its H1 receptor site, thereby preventing the vasodilatation, sneezing, and hypersecretion it causes. Decongestants may be helpful in reducing nasal obstruction through vasoconstriction, but the suitability of over-the-counter preparations for the younger child should be verified through the healthcare professional. Nasal corticosteroids are used to decrease inflammation in the nasal passages. For moderate to severe case of allergic rhinitis, leukotriene modifiers and mast cell stabilizers may be used. In children with more severe symptoms, immunotherapy may be used.

3. Carmella and Dominic need teaching about the condition, including the need to avoid offending allergens through environmental control (both at home and in school), such as using hypoallergenic covers on mattresses and pillows, washing bed linens in hot water weekly, removing clutter, eliminating stuffed toys, installing hardwood floors rather than carpeting, and avoiding exposure to chalk and strong odors in the classroom. Because it seems that Dominic has seasonal allergic rhinitis, Carmella also needs information about reducing Dominic's exposure to pollen (pollen counts are highest in the mornings between 5 and 10 AM). Other environmental measures to reduce allergen exposure should include wet-mop dusting, closing household windows at least during the allergy season, and frequently changing ventilation filters. One may be able to control exposure further by limiting household pets and making the home smoke free.

SECTION III: PRACTICING FOR NCLEX

Activity E CHOOSE THE BEST ANSWER.

1. c   2. a   3. b   4. d   5. c
6. c   7. b

CHAPTER 17

SECTION I: ASSESSING YOUR UNDERSTANDING

Activity A FILL IN THE BLANKS.

1. Hyponatremia
2. Hypernatremia
3. Hypokalemia
4. Hypophosphatemia
5. Hypercalcemia

Activity B MATCH THE FOLLOWING SIGNS OF DEHYDRATION WITH THE APPROPRIATE LEVEL OF DEHYDRATION. YOU MAY USE THE ANSWERS MORE THAN ONCE.

1. a, e   2. d   3. b, c

Activity C PUT IN ORDER THE SIGNS OF DEHYDRATION FROM MILD TO SEVERE IN TERMS OF CHANGES IN HEART RATE.

1. Mild: normal
2. Moderate: increased
3. Severe: increased

Activity D BRIEFLY ANSWER THE FOLLOWING.

1. The purpose of the arterial blood gases test is to measure acid–base imbalances.
2. The purpose of the urine specific gravity test measures the kidney's ability to dilute and concentrate urine.
3. Diet influences color; if passage is rapid, stool may be yellow or green
4. The nurse would look at ways to increase phosphorus in the diet or make sure the supplements are being administered.
5. Nursing responsibilities include monitoring serum calcium levels. Also, assess neuromuscular and cardiac status, maintain fluid balance, and provide parent teaching.

SECTION II: APPLYING YOUR KNOWLEDGE

Activity E CONSIDER THE SCENARIO AND ANSWER THE QUESTIONS.

1. Jamie is experiencing moderate dehydration and the symptoms in the scenario that identify this are decreased urine output; lethargy; 8% weight loss; his lips are dry; he is not producing tears; tachycardia is evident; he has a weak, thready pulse; and his skin temperature is cool.
2. The parent should be given information about administering oral rehydration therapy (ORT). Milk is not an appropriate source of rehydration and the parent should be instructed to use an ORT like Pedialyte instead. The parents should be instructed to give the ORT to replace 75 mL/kg over 4 hours, which would be the equivalent to about 1 oz every 10 minutes. After the child is hydrated, ORT should be stopped. This should take less than 48 hours. If the vomiting continues and Jamie continues to get more lethargic and shows signs of getting worse, the parent should call the doctor for possible IV fluid replacement.

SECTION III: PRACTICING FOR NCLEX

Activity F FILL IN THE BLANKS.

1. Hypermagnesemia
2. Hypomagnesemia
3. Hypercalcemia
4. Hyperkalemia
5. Potassium

Activity G CHOOSE THE BEST ANSWER.

1. **Answer: c**
   RATIONALE: Teaching the parents about dehydration prevention would be the first priority. IV fluids are used for moderate to severe dehydration. Antidiarrheal medication is usually contraindicated in children.

2. **Answer: a**
   RATIONALE: Children can continue losing fluids through insensible losses, which include sweating and breathing. Fluids are also lost through blood draws and urine, but this is not the only ways children lose fluids. Saliva is not a main source of fluid loss.

3. **Answer: d**
   RATIONALE: Infants' thirst mechanisms are not fully developed until they are older. The infant may have been so lethargic he or she could not have taken the bottle.

4. **Answer: a**
   RATIONALE: All body systems should be included in an assessment for fluid and electrolyte balance in a child. The skin integument and neurologic systems can also give indications about the child's fluid and electrolyte status.

5. **Answer: c**
   RATIONALE: The child's neurologic system is affected by dehydration. There is nothing in the history that indicates the child was experiencing pain or having respiratory difficulty.

6. **Answer: a**
   RATIONALE: Decreased blood pressure is a late sign of dehydration. This is not going to cause increased urinary output and the body is not compensating for the loss.

7. **Answer: a**
   RATIONALE: Encouraging oral fluid intake is the first intervention with dehydration. If the child is experiencing moderate or severe dehydration, then other methods may be used to replace the fluids lost.

8. **Answer: d**
   RATIONALE: It is important to watch for any signs of fever with a PICC line. This could be an indication of an infection related to the PICC line. The other symptoms are also important to watch for, but fever would be the most likely symptom related to the PICC line.

9. **Answer: b**
   RATIONALE: Administering less than the required amount is important for a child who may have a renal impairment. There is the potential for medication error as well, but this is not the most likely reason for the less-than-required amount.

10. **Answer: c**
    RATIONALE: Abnormal fluid losses are most likely the result of suctioning. Fluids are lost from this procedure.

CHAPTER 18

SECTION I: ASSESSING YOUR UNDERSTANDING

Activity A FILL IN THE BLANKS.

1. Fluid and electrolyte
2. Lactose
3. Meconium
4. Ostomy
5. Breast-feeding
6. Continuous enteral nutrition
7. Cleft lip
8. Intestinal atresia

Activity B MATCH THE BLOOD STUDY IN COLUMN A WITH ITS PURPOSE LISTED IN COLUMN B.

| 1. b | 2. e | 3. f | 4. c | 5. d |
| 6. g | 7. a | | | |

Activity C PLACE THE FOLLOWING PHYSICAL ASSESSMENT TECHNIQUES IN THE ORDER IN WHICH THEY SHOULD BE PERFORMED TO OBTAIN AN ACCURATE ASSESSMENT OF BOWEL SOUNDS.

Answer: a, d, b, c
   RATIONALE: The usual order of physical assessment techniques is altered during assessment of the abdomen. To obtain an accurate assessment of bowel sounds, auscultation must precede percussion and palpation.

Activity D BRIEFLY ANSWER THE FOLLOWING.

1. The four primary functions of the gastrointestinal system are ingestion, digestion, absorption of nutrients, and excretion of solid waste.
2. Activities involved in the care of the child receiving enteral nutrition include managing the enteral feeding tube and enteral nutrition delivery system to ensure accurate delivery of fluid and nutrients, and prevent system-related complications; monitoring the child's response to enteral nutrition, including metabolic complications; and supporting the child's and family's educational and developmental needs with regard to the therapy.

3. The nurse should teach the family (and child, as developmentally appropriate) how to care for the enteral feeding tube, to prepare and administer enteral feedings, to monitor for complications, and to attend to developmental and safety issues.

4. Malformations of the upper GI tract that can affect GI function include cleft lip, cleft palate, esophageal atresia, tracheoesophageal fistula, and pyloric stenosis.

5. Inflammatory disorders of the GI tract include gastroenteritis, appendicitis, inflammatory bowel disease, and pancreatitis. Gastroenteritis—inflammation of the GI tract—may be caused by gastrointestinal irritants such as bacteria, viruses, and toxins produced by fish, mushrooms, and chemicals (such as food additives). Appendicitis is an obstruction of the vermiform appendiceal lumen at the end of the cecum.

6. Possible causes of idiopathic acute pancreatitis include infections from bacteria or viral agents, medications, most commonly valproic acid, trauma, and gallstones or structural abnormalities.

7. Disorders of GI motility and function involve a diverse group of disorders that includes functional abdominal pain and irritable bowel syndrome (types of chronic abdominal pain), colic, gastroesophageal reflux disease, constipation, and encopresis.

8. After a positive diagnosis of functional abdominal pain or IBS is determined, education and reassurance of the child and parents are the key elements in the treatment plan. An interdisciplinary team approach is most beneficial for these complex problems. The physician, nurse, social worker, dietitian, and other healthcare professionals work with the family to outline the plan of care and goals. The nurse should reassure the child and family that the symptoms are not uncommon, and should explain the underlying mechanism of the abdominal pain.

Activity E CONSIDER THE SCENARIO AND ANSWER THE QUESTIONS.

1. The nurse should explain to Ella about the types of failure to thrive (FTT) that exist and make sure there is not an organic cause for Jakob's FTT. The nurse should stress that regardless of the etiology, FTT during the first year of life is a serious condition that may affect postnatal brain growth. The nurse should also explore possible nonorganic causes of FTT (such as depression, substance use, social isolation) with the mother, as well as possible infant behaviors contributing to the cause (such as being difficult to feed, apathetic, not wanting to be touched, and so forth).

2. The nurse should perform a careful history to direct the plan of care, which includes the prenatal history with regard to maternal lifestyle, medication use, and illnesses; birth history; postnatal history; and the reason for the current medical encounter.

The nurse should also verify the child's age to ensure that the child's growth parameters are plotted correctly on growth charts. When malnutrition or inadequate growth is established, a plan is developed to support the nutritional deficit while the workup for the etiology ensues. The nurse should explore the type of formula being used and its preparation, and ask for a typical recall of any solid foods the child is eating. The nurse must set up ongoing monitoring, with supportive interdisciplinary interventions from a physician, nurse, dietitian, medical social worker, occupational therapist, and child life specialist. Additional expertise, such as that of a psychologist or psychiatrist, may be indicated. It should be stated that providing adequate energy through calories for growth is the cornerstone of therapy for FTT. After the child has demonstrated a successful weight-gaining pattern, a follow-up plan is determined, and the interdisciplinary approach ensures that all aspects of community programs are accessed.

Activity F CHOOSE THE BEST ANSWER.

1. **Answer: b**
   RATIONALE: The nurse may demonstrate parts of the examination on a stuffed animal to help put Jason at ease and enhance cooperation. The nurse should not bribe him with candy; instead, the nurse could allow Jason to handle the examination tools so he is not afraid of them. Draping Jason would not calm him; however, adolescents should be draped to maintain privacy.

2. **Answer: c**
   RATIONALE: Stools with red blood and mucus are associated with intussusception. Stools commonly seen with cystic fibrosis are fatty stools. Stools associated with biliary atresia are clay colored, and stools indicating anal fissures have bright-red or maroon blood per rectum.

3. **Answer: a**
   RATIONALE: Emesis containing bright-red blood indicates acute upper GI bleeding. Emesis containing green or yellow bile indicates GI obstruction. Bright-red or maroon blood per rectum is usually associated with bleeding from the lower GI tract or anal fissures. Clay-colored stool occurs with biliary atresia or biliary tract obstruction.

4. **Answer: d**
   RATIONALE: The puree, mechanical soft diet is recommended for dysphagia and esophageal structure. High fiber is recommended for constipation and irritable bowel syndrome; high protein for weight control, wound healing, and cystic fibrosis; and fat is controlled for pancreatitis and gall bladder disease.

5. **Answer: b**
   RATIONALE: Rectobulbar urethral fistula is classified as intermediate, anocutaneous fistula is low, and

anorectal agenesis and rectal atresia are classified as high anorectal malformations.

6. Answer: d

RATIONALE: Gastroenteritis can be caused by microbes (bacteria, viruses, and parasites), by non-microbial food-borne agents found in certain types of fish and mushrooms, and by monosodium glutamate found in Chinese food.

7. Answer: d

RATIONALE: The presence of granulomas is more than 50% in Crohn's disease and is absent in ulcerative colitis. Fistulas or strictures are absent in ulcerative colitis and are present in Crohn's disease. Ulcerative colitis has shallow ulcerations limited to the mucosal and submucosal layers, and lesions are continuous and uniform. In Crohn's disease, ulcerations are transmural, penetrating all layers of GI tract, and lesions are intermittent.

8. Answer: c

RATIONALE: There are many causes of constipation in children, including excessive dairy intake, a diet low in fiber, starting toilet training too early, and malnutrition or underfeeding.

9. Answer: a

RATIONALE: Cirrhosis can be cause by certain infectious diseases, metabolic disorders (including cystic fibrosis), biliary malformations, toxic exposure, and others conditions, such as Parenteral Nutrition-Associated Liver Disease (PNALD) and neonatal hepatitis.

10. Answer: a

RATIONALE: Monitor the position of the G tube or G-J tube before each feeding and conduct site care by pulling back gently on the tube to ensure proper positioning. If the tube becomes dislodged, cover the site with clean gauze and tape, and notify the healthcare provider. Flush the tube with water after each intermittent feeding or every 4 to 6 hours during continuous feedings, per protocol. Administer medications in liquid form. If medications must be crushed, consult with a pharmacist regarding the appropriate solution for dissolving medications. Never crush enteric-coated or time-release medications.

Activity G CHOOSE ALL ANSWERS THAT APPLY.

1. Answer: a, b, c, d

RATIONALE: GI diseases that contribute to organic failure to thrive include gastroesophageal reflux disease, celiac disease, malabsorption syndromes, structural anomalies that affect oral motor function (e.g., cleft palate), tracheoesophageal fistula, pyloric stenosis, intractable diarrhea, Hirschsprung's disease, inflammatory bowel disease, and chronic liver disease (e.g., biliary atresia, hepatitis). Cerebral palsy is an neuromuscular disease and diabetes insipidus is an endocrine disease.

2. Answer: a, b, c

RATIONALE: X-rays are used to find obstructions, air and fluid levels, structural changes, and calcifications. Barium swallow and upper GI series detect structural abnormalities, foreign bodies, and so forth. Gastric emptying studies detect motility disorders. Liver biliary scans detect biliary atresia. Anorectal manometry diagnoses constipation, fecal incontinence, and dysmotility disorders.

3. Answer: a, b, e, f

RATIONALE: Immediate postoperative care focuses on airway management, hemostasis, and pain control. The child is at risk for airway compromise, and the use of a high-humidity oxygen tent may be ordered. The nurse should observe the child carefully for bleeding and excess mucus in the mouth, and place the child on her abdomen with the bed raised 30 degrees. The nurse should also administer pain medication as prescribed. Preoperative preparation of the family focuses on providing information regarding the surgical procedure and the child's postoperative care needs both in the hospital and at home.

CHAPTER 19

SECTION I: ASSESSING YOUR UNDERSTANDING

Activity A FILL IN THE BLANKS.

1. Renal replacement therapies
2. Urethritis
3. Secondary
4. DDAVP (desmopressin acetate)
5. Hypospadias

Activity B MATCH THE FOLLOWING THE TYPES OF DISORDERS IN COLUMN A WITH THE MOST LIKELY CLINICAL SIGNS IN COLUMN B. YOU MAY USE THE ANSWERS ONLY ONCE.

1. a   **2.** e   **3.** b   **4.** c   **5.** d

Activity C STARTING WITH GRADE 2, DESCRIBE EACH GRADE IN THE ORDER OF WHAT OCCURS IN VUR.

Grade II urine refluxes into the ureter and upper collecting system without dilatation. Grade III urine refluxes into a dilated ureter and upper collecting system with no or mild blunting of the calyces. Grade IV urine refluxes into a grossly dilated ureter and upper collecting system with moderate blunting of the calyces. Grade V urine refluxes into a massively dilated, tortuous ureter and upper collecting system with severe blunting of the calyces.

Activity D BRIEFLY ANSWER THE FOLLOWING.

1. The rudimentary kidney is formed during the first month of gestation and starts to produce urine by the 12th week. The placenta serves as a "pseudo kidney," helping regulate fluid and electrolyte balance. The kidneys do not function until after birth, and they do not reach maturity until age 2 years.
2. Human lymphocyte antigen (HLA) typing and serum crossmatch are used, along with having a compatible blood type.
3. Children with primary enuresis have never achieved continence. With secondary enuresis, the child achieves continence for at least 6 months, but then becomes incontinent again.
4. Scrotal palpation works well if the examiner has warm hands, and relaxation can be encouraged by placing the toddler in his parent's lap in the frog-leg position or cross-legged in the older boys. Applying pressure at the external inguinal ring will help isolate the testicle. A milking action to maneuver the testicle into the scrotal sac is used.
5. It is a condition resulting from forced retraction of the foreskin. This creates pain, distal edema, and difficulty replacing the foreskin. Emergency medical intervention is needed to relieve the obstruction.
6. Discuss the importance of administering oral antibiotics for the full course of therapy, obtaining a urine culture 48 to 72 hours after initiating treatment. Urine cultures should be checked every 3 months for a 1-year period, and a Voiding Cystourethrogram (VCUG) and renal ultrasound are common diagnostic procedures performed at this age to rule out other genitourinary conditions. Increase the patient's fluid intake and maintain proper hygiene. The child should avoid irritants such as bubble baths.

SECTION II: APPLYING YOUR KNOWLEDGE

Activity E CONSIDER THE SCENARIO AND ANSWER THE QUESTIONS.

1. This finding is consistent commonly with a varicocele. The teen should be told the doctor will probably order an ultrasound and these are not caused by a sexual activity.
2. This is usually treated by surgery. Most people have no problems after this is corrected by surgery and it should not affect future sexual activity. It is important the teen perform self-exams for reoccurrence of the problem.

SECTION III: PRACTICING FOR NCLEX

Activity F FILL IN THE BLANKS.

1. Hydronephrosis
2. Urethras
3. Latex
4. Hemodialysis
5. Pyelonephritis

Activity G CHOOSE THE BEST ANSWER.

1. **Answer: a**
   RATIONALE: The urine should be kept in the refrigerator to prevent false-positive results. It is not necessary to collect the urine in a catheter if the child is potty trained.
2. **Answer: c**
   RATIONALE: The stoma is a ureterostomy (detaches the ureter from the bladder and brings it to the surface of the abdomen), pyelostomy (creating an opening to the kidney pelvis), or vesicostomy (creating an opening to the bladder).
3. **Answer: c**
   RATIONALE: The age to teach a child self-catheterization depends on developmental and emotional factors, such as attention span, fine motor and manipulative control, family support, emotional readiness, and ability to perform sequential behaviors. Individualized judgment and procedural adaptation are required for children who are physically, emotionally, or developmentally challenged. Full independence with the procedure occurs when the child acquires a concept of time and record keeping, typically around age 6 to 8 years.
4. **Answer: a**
   RATIONALE: The most likely cause of the problem with how the catheter is functioning is constipation. The other symptoms listed would not cause the catheter to have a decrease in how it is functioning.
5. **Answer: b**
   RATIONALE: The parents should be taught this is a clean procedure. This is not considered a sterile procedure. The intermittent catheter should be performed on a routine basis. Performing it just morning and night or when the bladder is distended is not appropriate.
6. **Answer: a**
   RATIONALE: Peritonitis is a complication of peritoneal dialysis. The nurse should observe the patient for generalized abdominal pain and cloudy urine.
7. **Answer: a**
   RATIONALE: Parents should check for a bruit or feel for a thrill daily when a child has an arteriovenous fistula. The patency of this fistula and is extremely important to be checked.
8. **Answer: d**
   RATIONALE: HLA (human lymphocyte antigen) typing is performed to determine whether the child is compatible with another person for kidney donations. It examines the white blood cells for antigens involved in the immune response.
9. **Answer: b**
   RATIONALE: The child will need to be on antirejection medication for as long as he or she has the transplanted kidney. The other answers discuss taking the medication for a reduced period of time.

10. Answer: a

RATIONALE: If cystitis is left untreated, it can lead to pyelonephritis, which can in turn cause kidney damage and hypertension. Hydronephrosis is a condition in which urine backs up into the renal pelvis and calyces, which dilate and impair renal function and is not caused by cystitis. VUR is a congenital defect. *Escherichia coli* is a bacteria that actually can cause the cystitis.

CHAPTER 20

SECTION I: ASSESSING YOUR UNDERSTANDING

Activity A FILL IN THE BLANKS.

1. Boston
2. Logrolling
3. Subluxation
4. 40
5. Lordosis
6. Physes
7. Osteomyelitis

Activity B MATCH THE TERM IN COLUMN A WITH THE PROPER DEFINITION IN COLUMN B.

1. a   2. c   3. b   4. e   5. d

Activity C MATCH THE TYPE OF SPRAIN IN COLUMN A WITH THE DESCRIPTIVE PHRASE IN COLUMN B.

1. b   2. c   3. a

Activity D PLACE THE FOLLOWING STEPS IN THE PROPER SEQUENCE.

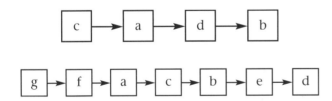

Activity E BRIEFLY ANSWER THE FOLLOWING.

1. Manual traction uses force applied to the bones by a physician, nurse, or technician to keep them in alignment. Skin traction is applied to the skin using skin adherents, Ace wraps, commercial traction tape, or special foam boots, to which the pull is applied. Skeletal fracture refers to any traction apparatus in which the pull force is applied directly to the skeleton via pins, wires, screws, and/or tongs that are inserted into the appropriate area of bone.

2. When holding the infant's heel in one hand, try to position the foot to midline with the other hand. If you are able to straighten the foot, the child has metatarsus adductus, not clubfoot.

3. All types of osteomyelitis can cause massive bone destruction and life-threatening sepsis.

4. The classic sign of compartment syndrome is unrelenting pain that is not relieved by narcotics.

SECTION II: APPLYING YOUR KNOWLEDGE

Activity F CONSIDER THE SCENARIO AND ANSWER THE QUESTIONS.

1. It would be important to tell the mother that developmental dysplasia of the hip (DDH) is one of the most common defects in the newborn infant, and it is more common in girls, breech deliveries, and in those with a familial history. Anita should be reassured that nothing she did or did not do during her pregnancy caused this condition, and that it is fairly common and treatable.

2. A careful birth history should be assessed, including type of birth and whether the baby was breech. These would be indicators to potential risk of DDH. In the newborn infant, the Ortolani and Barlow tests are performed to assess for dislocation. The nurse should observe for leg length discrepancy, restricted or diminished motion, or limited abduction on the affected side. Eight to 12 weeks after birth, the Ortolani and Barlow tests are no longer valid, and other assessments should be performed. In the 3-month-old infant, limited adduction of the affected hip is the predominate sign when the hip becomes fixed in the dislocated position. Asymmetric thigh folds and positive Galeazzi sign (one femur shorter than the other when measured with the hips and knees flexed) are physical findings that may be an indication of acetabulum abnormalities.

3. Preoperatively, the parents will need to be taught how the cast will position the child's hips and legs. Caring for a child in a cast, as well as handling, positioning, and moving the child, should be taught. Because skin breakdown is a major risk factor, the cast must be used in conjunction with moleskin. The parent must be taught how to keep the cast clean and dry. Bathing, dressing, and transporting a child with a spica cast must also be addressed. The parent should also be taught how to apply and remove the Pavlik harness. A return demonstration prior to discharge is necessary to ensure that the parent is comfortable with the procedure. How to perform activities of daily living, especially diaper changing, must be taught and demonstrated. Skin care must again be addressed.

SECTION III: PRACTICING FOR NCLEX

Activity G **CHOOSE THE BEST ANSWER.**

1. **Answer: b**

   RATIONALE: The body responds to the change in blood volume, anesthetic medications, and physical and emotional stress of the surgical procedure by releasing ADH to hold on to fluids. Thus, the first indicator of SIADH is a decrease in urine output.

2. **Answer: b**

   RATIONALE: Because this boy is most concerned about the brace and perceives scoliosis as a girl's disease, putting the child in contact with someone undergoing the same problem would be helpful. The other suggestions could be helpful by engaging the boy's input in his treatment or reminding him that boys have less progression, but do not address his specific concerns.

3. **Answer: a**

   RATIONALE: Before discharge, the nurse must teach the family about administering the child's medication properly. The nurse must clearly indicate that the child should not miss a dose and must take all the medicine for the antibiotic therapy to be effective. It would be unhelpful to tell the parents that he may develop osteomyelitis, because they are already feeling guilty about not seeking medical attention. Avoiding constipation and recognizing fever and increasing pain are important, but the focus needs to be on teaching the family about proper medication administration for their child.

4. **Answer: c**

   RATIONALE: An electric blanket that is timed to turn on 1 hour before the girl awakens is an inexpensive, simple approach that can be instituted immediately. A warm bath every morning would likely be impractical in a home with four school-aged children. Paraffin baths would only benefit the small joints of the hands, not generalized body stiffness. A waterbed would be helpful to ease stiffness, but may be impractical as a result of space and budgetary constraints.

5. **Answer: d**

   RATIONALE: Suggesting a support group with other girls undergoing steroid therapy for systemic lupus erythematosus (SLE) would be most helpful to boost self-esteem and encourage independence. Telling her that weight gain is common, and referring to facial fullness would be unhelpful and could increase her sensitivity. Simply handing her a pamphlet would be unhelpful. Reminding her to take her medicine to avoid an acute episode is true, but may be perceived as threatening and will not address the underlying issues.

6. **Answer: b**

   RATIONALE: Lack of swelling at the fracture site of a young child would indicate osteogenesis imperfecta (OI). Multiple fractures and bruising of the affected arm are findings consistent with both abuse and OI. A spiral fracture would be less likely to occur in a small child and is more indicative of abuse and does not necessarily point to OI.

7. **Answer: a**

   RATIONALE: It is common for parents to hear the word *surgery* and subsequently "tune out" the rest of the information presented by the physician. It is important for the nurse to restate the fact that less than 1% of children actually need surgery. Telling the parents that the anteversion usually resolves by age 9 is correct, but this does not address their fears about surgery. Additional facts about the time frame and recovery period for the surgery would be unnecessary at this time.

8. **Answer: b**

   RATIONALE: Telling the mother that there are home healthcare services and other community agencies available to help with her son's treatment and care would likely ensure compliance, reduce her resistance, and ease her mind. Telling her that her son could have permanent difficulties without treatment is true, but does not offer solutions. Telling her that she can learn about traction and immobilization would likely intimidate her, and, as a working mother, it is impractical for her to be his sole caregiver. Making a reference to home tutoring only addresses his educational needs.

9. **Answer: b**

   RATIONALE: It is most important to keep the boy's shoe in place to help control swelling and until any fractures are ruled out by x-rays.

10. **Answer: d**

    RATIONALE: The best course of action would be distraction and offering the school-aged child some control. Inviting the girl to select the color of her cast will take her mind off of her fear and relax her. The other comments are appropriate, but distraction and a feeling of some control would be best in this situation.

Activity H **CHOOSE ALL ANSWERS THAT APPLY.**

1. **Answer: b, c, d, f**

   RATIONALE: Encouraging the child to participate in care decisions is a psychosocial intervention. Using serial manipulation restores joint mobility and assessing for skin breakdown minimizes complications of immobility. Assisting the child to perform range-of-motion exercises twice daily and allowing the child to perform tasks at his or her own rate while also encouraging and facilitating early ambulation and other age-appropriate activities of daily living maximizes mobility.

2. **Answer: a, b, d, e**

   RATIONALE: CBC evaluates several indicators, including infection and anemia. CRP measures a protein in the blood that is released when infection is present. Calcium and phosphorous levels assist in diagnosing renal and skeletal diseases. Erythrocyte sedimentation rates indicate the presence of an inflammatory process. Blood culture and sensitivity diagnose bacteremia or septicemia, and arthrography visualizes selected joints for injuries or abnormalities.

3. **Answer: b, e, f**
   RATIONALE: Aspirating fluid from the joints determines cause and type of joint disorder, and effusion. Increased or abnormal levels possibly indicate noninflammatory abnormalities (e.g., traumatic arthritis), inflammatory abnormalities (e.g., rheumatoid arthritis, systemic lupus erythematosus), septic abnormalities (e.g., septic arthritis), or hemorrhagic abnormalities.

4. **Answer: a, d, e**
   RATIONALE: Foods high in phosphorous include milk, cheese, egg yolks, meat, fish, nuts, whole-grain cereals, and legumes.

5. **Answer: b, c, f**
   RATIONALE: According to the Salter-Harris classification, in a type II epiphyseal fracture there is fracture separation of the epiphysis, circulation remains intact, and growth is usually not affected.

CHAPTER 21

SECTION I: ASSESSING YOUR UNDERSTANDING

Activity A FILL IN THE BLANKS.

1. Synaptogenesis
2. Craniotomy
3. Disuse
4. Sequelae
5. Compensation
6. Dehydration
7. Decorticate

Activity B MATCH THE HEADACHE TYPE IN COLUMN A WITH THE PROPER ETIOLOGY IN COLUMN B.

1. c   **2.** d   **3.** a   **4.** e   **5.** f
6. b

Activity C MATCH CHARACTERISTICS IN COLUMN I WITH EITHER BREATH HOLDING (COLUMN A) OR SEIZURE (COLUMN B) BY PLACING A MARK IN THE APPROPRIATE COLUMN.

1. a   **2.** b   **3.** a   **4.** a   **5.** b
6. b   **7.** a, b   **8.** b   **9.** a   **10.** b

Activity D PLACE THE FOLLOWING IN THE PROPER ORDER.

1.

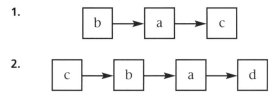

2.

Activity E BRIEFLY ANSWER THE FOLLOWING.

1. A comprehensive neurologic assessment includes health history and evaluation of mental status, behavior, achievement of developmental milestones, motor and sensory functions, infant reflexes, cranial nerve function, and deep tendon reflexes.

2. The primary elements of nursing care for a child with increased ICP include monitoring for changes in neurologic function and assessing ICP; performing rapid intervention if neurologic deterioration occurs; maintaining the integrity of the monitoring system, assessing the child for signs of infection, hemorrhage, or CSF leakage; and reducing the child's pain, crying, and agitation with comfort measures, including the timely use of analgesics and sedatives as necessary.

3. Promote optimal cerebral perfusion, avoid airway compromise, respond to altered sensorium and changes in level of consciousness, prevent infection, and facilitate rehabilitation and home care.

4. Prevent infection, neurologic injury, and injury to the limbs secondary to disuse. Promote optimal bowel and bladder function. Assess skin integrity. Assist with determining the child's functional abilities, including motor performance and sensory deficits. Promote family coping and the child's positive self-concept.

5. Ask about any history of trauma, CNS infection, familial megalencephaly, birth injury, or prematurity, and note the onset and duration of symptoms. Measure head circumference; note spilt sutures or a full or bulging fontanel, especially one that is nonpulsatile, indicating high pressure. Note other clinical signs and symptoms that become apparent as hydrocephalus progresses, including "sunset appearance," Collier's sign, prominent scalp veins, lethargy, irritability, high-pitched cry, and projectile vomiting.

SECTION II: APPLYING YOUR KNOWLEDGE

Activity F CONSIDER THE SCENARIO AND ANSWER THE QUESTIONS.

1. The nurse should explain to the parents that treating many neurosurgical injuries requires direct access to the brain through the bony structures of the skull, and a craniotomy involves creating a "flap" opening of the skill in which the bone is removed and then replaced at the completion of surgery. In Paul's case, it is the physician's priority to obtain informed consent from the parents by discussing the purpose of the surgery, the possibility of alternative treatment or lack of treatment, the potential risks, and the expected outcomes. The nurse should be present to reinforce and clarify the information presented in the discussion.

2. Parents are often overwhelmed with fear and anxiety when faced with the prospect of brain surgery for their child. The nurse should provide emotional support throughout the entire process. Because neurosurgical procedures often involve the head and face, the nurse should be aware that some of the preoperative anxiety and fear may be related to shaving the hair and worrying about visible scars. The nurse should prepare the family for postoperative effects of surgery, and be available to support the family and listen to them as they express their feelings about the events.

3. The nurse should perform an accurate, well-documented preoperative neurologic baseline assessment to accurately track postoperative functioning and monitor for potential complications. The nursing role after cranial surgery involves frequent acute neurologic monitoring and assessment of vital signs, intake and output, dressing, drainage, and pain to monitor the child for any potential complications. The nurse should be aware that the possibility of CSF drainage is greater when the surgery is done after a traumatic injury like Paul sustained.

SECTION III: PRACTICING FOR NCLEX

Activity G CHOOSE THE BEST ANSWER.

1. **Answer: b**
   RATIONALE: Applying elbow splints to prevent the child from touching the incision is the most valuable intervention postoperatively. Reviewing before-and-after photos educates the parents preoperatively. Hard-shell helmets are a nonsurgical alternative. Orbital edema, which may cause the child's eyes to swell shut, is common with this surgery.

2. **Answer: a**
   RATIONALE: It is important to avoid over hydration to prevent the onset of SIADH; fluids are often restricted for this reason. Droplet precautions are necessary only until 24 hours of effective antibiotic therapy have elapsed. Pain can be managed, but probably not eliminated. Administer antibiotics as soon as meningitis is suspected.

3. **Answer: c**
   RATIONALE: After surgical excision and drainage of the abscess, or if surgery is not necessary, parents can be taught to complete the course of antibiotics at home. Lumbar puncture is contraindicated with brain abscesses. There is no risk of contagion with brain abscesses. Monitoring to avoid respiratory distress is a necessary intervention for Chiari malformation, not brain abscess.

4. **Answer: d**
   RATIONALE: The incubation time for tetanus is 7 to 14 days. If the child did not care for the camping injury properly, it could have caused infection. Frequent vomiting is not a symptom of tetanus. DT vaccinations must be updated every 5 years

to be effective. The home accident probably received proper care.

5. **Answer: c**
   RATIONALE: The child is at risk for joint contractures, skin breakdown, and deep vein thromboses. These complications can be minimized by performing passive motion exercises, frequent repositioning, and meticulous skin care. The disease has a good prognosis for most children. Monitoring for change in ICP is not indicated for this disease. Guillain-Barré is caused by a viral illness, making antibiotics unnecessary.

6. **Answer: a**
   RATIONALE: With a mild concussion, a patient who did not lose consciousness, sustain any other injuries, and is acting normally can be sent home. The nurse should summarize concisely how to care for the child. Being insistent or confrontational may antagonize the parents and they may not receive valuable information, but the nurse must attempt to educate the parents regarding signs and symptoms that would indicate a problem.

7. **Answer: b**
   RATIONALE: All children younger than 3 and any child whose head size is questionable should have their head circumference measured and plotted on a growth chart. At this point, there is no need to determine the mother's knowledge of hydrocephalus or to educate her about head size changes. There would be no need to assess the child's level of consciousness either.

8. **Answer: a**
   RATIONALE: Monitoring fluid and electrolyte status closely to avoid fluid overload and resulting edema is most effective for this client. Rectal diazepam would not be appropriate for this child because of age. The parents would not need support for anticipatory grieving. Letting the child listen to favorite music may be too stimulating.

9. **Answer: a**
   RATIONALE: The prognosis for febrile seizures is generally good, and children rarely have any short- or long-term deficits. Diagnostic evaluation of a child who presents with a seizure associated with fever is aimed at determining whether the child had a febrile seizure or if a more serious, underlying condition is present. For the child who has a history of febrile seizures, using daily antiepileptic medication to prevent further seizure is not recommended, because the medication causes substantial adverse effects. Rectal diazepam is often recommended for emergency treatment of febrile seizures and is indicated for children with a history of prolonged or multiple febrile seizures, and for those who live long distances from medical care.

10. **Answer: c**
    RATIONALE: It is important to let the client know how he became infected. This way he may take precautions against infection and tell others to do

the same. Trying to frighten an adolescent will probably make him less receptive to further information. Describing the physiology of the infection or the cause of the headache should be reserved until the client asks about it.

Activity H CHOOSE ALL ANSWERS THAT APPLY.

1. **Answer: a, c, f**
   RATIONALE: The nurse should allow ICP to return to baseline between nursing activities and plan nursing care to provide rest periods. Environmental stimuli should be decreased and anticonvulsants administered as appropriate. The patient should be positioned with the head of the bed up 30 degrees or more and fluids should be restricted. The nurse should perform passive range-of-motion exercises to prevent rigidity of the muscles.
2. **Answer: a, b, f**
   RATIONALE: The nurse should note widening pulse pressure, bradycardia, and altered respirations (Cushing's triad) and report immediately, and maintain a neutral position of the head and neck. Palpating infant fontanels is recommended to assess the neurologic system. Fluids should be restricted per prescriber's order and a daily stool softener should be given to reduce hard stools or straining. Deep breathing exercises should be encouraged.
3. **Answer: a, b, c**
   RATIONALE: After a seizure, the nurse should position the child in a side-lying position with the head in the midline position and should not hyperextend the neck. The nurse should allow the seizure to end without interference and should remove any eyeglasses to prevent injury. Clothing should be loosened and nothing should be placed in the child's mouth.
4. **Answer: a, b, e, f**
   RATIONALE: Symptoms of myasthenia crisis include anoxia, cyanosis, bowel and bladder incontinence, decreased urinary output, absence of swallow reflex, and cough. Symptoms of cholinergic crisis include anticholinergic drug toxicity, hypotension, nausea, vomiting, diarrhea, abdominal cramps, pallor, blurred vision, and facial muscle twitching.

CHAPTER 22

SECTION I: ASSESSING YOUR UNDERSTANDING

Activity A FILL IN THE BLANKS.

1. Cancer
2. Multimodal
3. Hodgkin's disease
4. 5
5. Radiation

Activity B MATCH TERMS ASSOCIATED WITH CANCER CHEMOTHERAPY IN COLUMN A WITH THE DEFINITION LISTED IN COLUMN B.

1. b   2. d   3. a   4. c   5. e

Activity C PLACE THE FOLLOWING STAGES OF CHEMOTHERAPY IN THE ORDER IN WHICH THEY ARE INITIATED IN THE PROCESS.

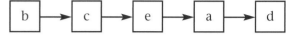

b → c → e → a → d

Activity D BRIEFLY ANSWER THE FOLLOWING.

1. Cancers in children differ substantially from cancers in adults. Most childhood cancers arise from the embryonic mesodermal germ layer, and as a result, 92% of childhood cancers (sarcomas, leukemias, and lymphomas) develop from primitive embryonal tissue. The remaining 8% of childhood cancers arise from neuroectodermal tissue and give rise to central nervous system (CNS) tumors (Ruccione, 2004). In contrast, most adult cancers involve the epithelial tissue and are called *carcinomas*. Epithelial cancers are quite rare in children younger than 15 years.
2. The signs and symptoms of cancer in children are primarily the result of one or more of the following factors:
   - Compression, infiltration, or obstruction caused by the tumor
   - Changes in blood cell production, such as decreased hemoglobin, hematocrit, white blood count, or platelets
   - Secretion of a substance by the tumor that interferes with normal organ functioning
   - Metabolic, electrolyte, hormonal, or immunologic alterations caused by tumor metabolism or cell death
3. A stage III rhabdomyosarcoma is a localized tumor with gross residual disease after incomplete removal or biopsy only.
4. Nursing responsibilities for the child receiving radiation therapy include providing concrete explanations to the child and the child's family regarding the radiation procedure and its side effects, preparing the child for the treatment, and managing the side effects of the therapy and preventing further complications.
5. The exact mechanism of action of BRMs is unclear. However, they apparently can modify the immune response to the cancer, act directly against the tumor by suppressing tumor growth or killing the tumor cell, and alter other biologic factors that can directly or indirectly influence the viability of the tumor (McCune, 2008, p. 109).

6. Stressors related to a cancer diagnosis include, but are not limited to
   - The shock of the diagnosis of cancer
   - Role changes necessary to meet the demands of caring for a chronically ill child
   - The financial burden caused by medical costs and a possible loss of income because it may be necessary for one parent to stay home with the child
   - Fear of losing the child
   - Marital discord
   - Feelings of guilt related to spending less time with the siblings and with one's spouse
   - The need to learn technical and medical information to better understand the child's disease and its treatment

SECTION II: APPLYING YOUR KNOWLEDGE

Activity E   CONSIDER THE SCENARIO AND ANSWER THE QUESTIONS.

1. Enlarged lymph nodes that are firm and painful on palpation and that are associated with weight loss, fever, and an abnormal chest x-ray may indicate a lymphoma, such as Hodgkin's disease or non-Hodgkin's lymphoma (NHL).

2. The nurse caring for Megan and her father should offer support and guidance as they undergo the tests for cancer. The nurse should be familiar with the procedures and the usual sequence in which they are conducted. The nurse should also establish an open, caring nurse–child relationship by giving simple, honest answers to Megan's questions and ensuring her safety during the tests by preventing or minimizing pain from the procedure or from the cancer itself. An age-appropriate explanation of what is being done and why will help ensure cooperation from Megan, and giving her freedom of movement (without being restrained) will help her feel she has some control over the situation.

3. The nurse could advocate for Megan and her father by looking into community services that may help with the medical bills and home care that may be necessary with a diagnosis of cancer. The nurse should also act as a coordinator of care and services provided to this family by arranging for appointments and providing referrals as needed. The home care nurse conducts ongoing assessments of the family's ability to care for the ill child in the home, assists in the procurement of medical equipment and supplies, provides needed healthcare interventions, and coordinates the delivery of home care services by other members of the team. Collaboration with the home care pharmacist, primary oncologist, physical and occupational therapist, nutritionist, speech therapist, and respiratory therapist is essential to ensure that all aspects of the child's development are supported.

SECTION III: PRACTICING FOR NCLEX

Activity F   CHOOSE THE BEST ANSWER.

1. **Answer: a**
   RATIONALE: Asymmetry of facial features may indicate a retinoblastoma or nasopharyngeal rhabdomyosarcoma.

2. **Answer: c**
   RATIONALE: The presence of pallor, ecchymoses, and petechiae may indicate that the cancer has invaded the bone marrow and is interrupting the normal production of red blood cells and platelets, as in leukemia. Enlarged lymph nodes may indicate Hodgkin's disease. Asymmetry of an extremity may indicate a bone tumor or soft-tissue sarcoma. Answer d is not true.

3. **Answer: b**
   RATIONALE: To prepare a patient for a lumbar puncture, the nurse should encourage fluids before and after LP, and empty the bladder before LP, because the child must remain supine for 4 to 6 hours after the procedure. In addition, premedicate for pain and maintain strict asepsis.

4. **Answer: d**
   RATIONALE: Increased WBC with the presence of lymphoblasts can indicate leukemia. A decreased neutrophil count indicates neutropenia. Decreased RBCs or Hgb or HB are seen in anemia. A platelet count less than $1,000,000/mm^3$ indicates thrombocytopenia.

5. **Answer: a**
   RATIONALE: Aspirated bone marrow is used for microscopic examination of cell type and morphology. This test is performed to determine when leukemia is present, if the tumor has spread to the bone marrow, or when a CBC suggests malfunctioning bone marrow.

6. **Answer: b**
   RATIONALE: Bruising or swelling around the eyes (proptosis) may indicate a soft-tissue mass. Pallor of the gums may indicate anemia. Enlarged or tender cervical lymph nodes may indicate lymphadenopathy. The presence of white reflection in the pupil of the eye may indicate retinoblastoma.

7. **Answer: c**
   RATIONALE: Adolescents should return to school as soon as possible after an illness or hospitalization. Parents should encourage usual activities and use the school reentry program to educate peers about the child's condition. Parents should not encourage adolescents to be overly dependent on nurses and family for physical care.

8. **Answer: b**
   RATIONALE: The common clinical presentation of Burkitt's lymphoma is abdominal primary, tumor lysis syndrome (increased uric acid and lactate dehydrogenase), jaw tumor (African), and propensity for spreading to bone marrow and the central nervous system. Tumor burden may be massive.

9. **Answer: d**
   RATIONALE: Patients with brain stem glioma present with the characteristic triad of signs and symptoms arising from early interference with the functioning of the cranial nerve nuclei, pyramidal tracts, and cerebellar pathways.

10. **Answer: a**
    RATIONALE: Interventions for tumor lysis syndrome include providing IV hydration, administering diuretics, administering allopurinol or rasburicase, monitoring serum chemistry levels, using oral and IV solutions specific to electrolyte needs, monitoring intake and output, and providing dialysis if renal failure occurs.

Activity G CHOOSE ALL ANSWERS THAT APPLY.

1. **Answer: b, c, f**
   RATIONALE: Child cancers are rare—2% of all cancers—and involve tissue instead of organs. Child cancers are usually nonepithelial, as opposed to adult cancers, which are usually epithelial carcinomas. Child cancers have a short period from initiation as opposed to those of adults, which have a long period. Adult cancers have a strong relationship to the environment. Child cancers are very responsive to chemotherapy, whereas adult cancers are less responsive.

2. **Answer: a, b, c, d**
   RATIONALE: Signs of septic shock include fever or hypothermia, tachycardia, tachypnea, peripheral vasodilation, leukocytosis, leucopenia, reduced mental alertness, and organ failure.

3. **Answer: a, c, e**
   RATIONALE: A patient with infratentorial tumors (brain stem and cerebellar) displays increased intracranial pressure, ataxia (gait, truncal), nystagmus, head tilt, diplopia, cranial nerve deficits, hypotonia, abnormal reflexes, changes in speech, hemiparesis, and a positive Babinski sign.

Activity H FILL IN THE BLANKS.

1. Bone marrow, peripheral, cord
2. Autologous, allogeneic

CHAPTER 23

SECTION I: ASSESSING YOUR UNDERSTANDING

Activity A FILL IN THE BLANKS.

1. Essential elements, waste products
2. Hemostasis
3. Stem cell
4. Polycythemia
5. Hematuria, hematemesis, hematochezia
6. Iron, folic acid

7. Intrinsic pathway
8. Coagulopathy

Activity B MATCH THE DISORDERS OF HEMOSTASIS LISTED IN COLUMN A WITH THEIR DEFINITIONS IN COLUMN B.

1. f	2. h	3. d	4. i	5. a
6. j	7. e	8. b	9. g	10. c

Activity C PLACE THE FOLLOWING IN THEIR PROPER ORDER OF OCCURRENCE.

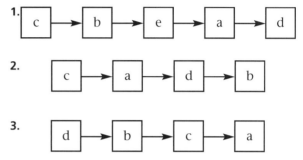

1. c → b → e → a → d
2. c → a → d → b
3. d → b → c → a

Activity D BRIEFLY ANSWER THE QUESTIONS.

1. Hematopoiesis depends on the stem cell for two major reasons: (1) The stem cell can differentiate to form progenitor (precursor) cells for red blood cells, white blood cells, and platelets; and (2) the stem cell is capable of self-renewal, providing a continuous supply of the cells required for hematopoiesis. Fetal blood and umbilical cord blood are rich sources of stem cells.

2. The erythrocyte (red blood cell) undergoes several developmental changes as it progresses through the prenatal period to infancy and childhood. These changes include shifts in production rate, life span, appearance, and type of hemoglobin (the erythrocyte's oxygen-carrying molecule).

3. Common types of crisis events associated with sickle cell disease include vasoocclusive crises, infections, acute splenic sequestration, and aplastic crises.

4. Interventions for the patient with iron deficiency anemia include, but are not limited to, teaching about the manifestations of the conditions (inadequate iron, decreased hemoglobin in red blood cells, decreased oxygenation of body tissues), informing about the causes of iron deficiency anemia (inadequate iron intake, especially during times of rapid physical growth; malabsorption of iron; iron loss related to excessive bleeding), educating about dietary sources of iron, and teaching about iron supplements, when prescribed.

5. Factors that may precipitate sickling of red blood cells include
   ■ Infection
   ■ Dehydration

- Hot and/or humid environment
- Cold air and/or water temperature
- High altitude
- Excessive physical activity

6. Goals of a chronic transfusion therapy program for children with severe chronic anemia include

- Maintain an Hb S level between 30% to 50% in children with sickle cell disease
- Provide primary stroke prevention or prevent stroke recurrence
- Treat chronic debilitating pain, pulmonary hypertension, and anemia associated with chronic renal failure
- Increase the quality of life for children with chronic heart failure
- Delay the onset of splenomegaly with hypersplenism and the accompanying need for splenectomy

---

SECTION II: APPLYING YOUR KNOWLEDGE

Activity E CONSIDER THE SCENARIO AND ANSWER THE QUESTIONS.

1. Incorporating the use of an interdisciplinary professional team that is affiliated with a center for comprehensive treatment of pediatric hematologic disorders is a key intervention. The nurse should ensure that the team collaborates with healthcare providers in the home community to provide complete care for Jabir. The team also must be aware of and follow the heath supervision guidelines recommended by the American Academy of Pediatrics (AAP, 2002), emphasizing the importance of an ongoing health maintenance program to manage sickle cell disease effectively. Jabir should have regular visits to the healthcare center to update the health history and physical assessment data, and to acquire needed interventions.

2. An important element of the teaching process is to assess the family's understanding of the child's home care needs and its ability to provide them. Management of sickle cell disease requires attention to the psychosocial needs of the child and the family. The nurse should assess the child's readiness to learn more about sickle cell disease, as well as the need to correct misperceptions that the child and family may have about the disorder, its effect, its complications, and its management. The teaching should also reflect the child's specific developmental needs as they change with developmental milestones. A concerted effort should be made to help Jabir develop effective coping skills for dealing with both physical and psychosocial concerns.

SECTION III: PRACTICING FOR NCLEX

Activity F CHOOSE THE BET ANSWER.

1. **Answer: a**
   RATIONALE: Hemoglobin F, composed of alpha and gamma globin chains, is the predominant hemoglobin during the fetal stage of development and at birth. An excess of hemoglobin F may be associated with hemoglobinopathies, such as sickle cell disease and certain other disorders.

2. **Answer: c**
   RATIONALE: Tachycardia and hypotension are associated with loss of blood in bleeding disorders, decreased hemoglobin level in anemias, and fever and infection in neutropenia.

3. **Answer: c**
   RATIONALE: Reduced platelet numbers identify thrombocytopenia. Decreases in RBC number, size, and hemoglobin content identify anemias. Increased WBC number and distribution identify infection; decreased granulocytes and WBC suggest neutropenia.

4. **Answer: d**
   RATIONALE: The Coombs' test detects antibodies attached to red blood cells. Antibody presence helps detect hemolytic disease of the newborn.

5. **Answer: a**
   RATIONALE: The nurse assisting with a total iron binding capacity (TIBC) and transferrin test should ensure that the child is fasting in the morning (circadian rhythm affects iron) prior to the lab draw, have a sample drawn before the child is given therapeutic iron or blood transfusion, and keep in mind that iron determinations in children who have had blood transfusions should be delayed for at least 4 days.

6. **Answer: a**
   RATIONALE: Assessing the child's tissue perfusion including skin color, warmth, pulses, capillary refill, complaints of numbness or tingling of extremities, vital signs, and oral mucosa indicates fluid balance, level of hydration, and effectiveness of fluid replacement.

7. **Answer: a**
   RATIONALE: Measures to prevent transfusion reactions include priming the infusion line with normal saline to decrease risk of hemolysis of red blood cells, monitoring the prescribed flow rate of infusion, using an infusion pump to regulate the flow, administering slowly during the first 15 minutes of infusion for all children, and remaining with the child during the first 15 to 30 minutes of transfusion, because most reactions occur during the first 30 minutes.

8. **Answer: b**
   RATIONALE: The nurse should encourage the child to progress from passive range-of-motion to active exercises as tolerated. Pain is better managed if it is not allowed to escalate. Anything placed in the

rectum may cause tearing and bleeding of the anal mucosa. Ibuprofen decreases the ability of the blood to clot.

9. **Answer: b**
   RATIONALE: Foods high in iron include liver, other red meats, clams, oysters, lima and navy beans, dark-green leafy vegetables, and dried fruit.

10. **Answer: d**
    RATIONALE: Fresh frozen plasma (FFP) is used for replacement of noncellular coagulation factors. Packed red blood cells (PRBCs) are used for symptomatic anemia and replacement therapy (e.g., during surgery). Platelets are used for bleeding associated with thrombocytopenia or platelet dysfunction.

11. **Answer: c**
    RATIONALE: Signs of a hemolytic reaction include fever, chills, urticaria, restlessness, headache, chest pain, tachycardia, hypotension, abdominal/lower back pain, oliguria, and shock.

Activity G **CHOOSE ALL ANSWERS THAT APPLY.**

1. **Answer: a, c, d, f**
   RATIONALE: Fever may be present with infections related to neutropenia. Fatigue, pallor, inadequate weight gain, and unexplained weight loss are common signs of anemia. Bleeding, bruising, and petechiae are signs of thrombocytopenias, ITP (low platelet count), and bleeding disorders. Jaundiced sclera can be present with hemolytic anemias, sickle cell disease, and thalassemia. Joint and muscle swelling is a sign of hemophilia. Lower extremity ulcers may be indications of an anemia.

2. **Answer: a, b, e, f**
   RATIONALE: Chronic complications of sickle cell anemia include skin ulcerations, vascular changes in the eyes, increased cardiac output, high liver enzyme levels, hyposthenuria, and chronic lung disease, to name a few.

3. **Answer: a, b, c**
   RATIONALE: Signs of an acute splenic sequestration include left upper quadrant abdominal pain and vomiting; decreased hemoglobin, hematocrit (number and size of red blood cells), and platelet count; increased reticulocyte count; and the presence of nucleated red blood cells.

Activity H **PLACE THE FOLLOWING EVENTS IN THE ORDER IN WHICH HEMOSTASIS OCCURS AFTER THE LOSS OF VASCULAR INTEGRITY.**

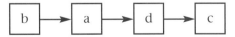

CHAPTER 24

SECTION I: ASSESSING YOUR UNDERSTANDING

Activity A **BRIEFLY ANSWER THE FOLLOWING.**

1. The three most common tick-borne infections are Rocky Mountain spotted fever, human monocytotropic ehrlichiosis, and Lyme disease.

2. The incubation period for pertussis is 7 to 10 days, during which the child is most contagious. The catarrhal phase occurs during this initial incubation period, producing coldlike symptoms (runny nose, scratchy throat, and mild cough). This stage is followed by the paroxysmal phase, characterized by periods of paroxysmal coughing, during which the child coughs violently, vomits, has apneic spells, and becomes cyanotic. At the end of the coughing attack, the patient gasps (whoops) for air. Infants younger than 6 months may not exhibit classic whooping. These intense spells of coughing often interfere with feeding and sleep. The paroxysmal phase lasts 2 to 6 weeks and is followed by a convalescent stage characterized by a persistent (but not paroxysmal) cough.

3. Transmission of CMV is by direct contact with virus-containing secretions, such as urine or saliva. This contact can occur in daycare centers or nurseries when drooling, teething babies share toys that they bite or gum. Adolescents may acquire CMV through sexual intercourse and kissing (saliva). Transmission from an infected mother to her infant may occur by transplacental passage of the virus in utero, passage of the neonate through an infected birth canal, or ingestion of infected breast milk. Other modes of transmission include blood transfusions and solid organ transplants.

4. Symptoms of mononucleosis present as a triad: sore throat (exudative pharyngitis), fever, and lymphadenopathy.

5. Two types of streptococci cause disease: group A and group B. Group A streptococcal (GAS) disease is one of the most common diseases of childhood, causing a variety of cutaneous and systemic infections and complications, with variable severity and prognosis. Group B streptococcus (GBS) is a leading cause of neonatal sepsis and death. Group B streptococci are gram-positive, aerobic diplococci.

Activity B **FILL IN THE BLANKS.**

1. Passive
2. Infectious
3. Pertussis
4. Mononucleosis
5. Measles

SECTION II: APPLYING YOUR KNOWLEDGE

Activity C **CONSIDER THE SCENARIO AND ANSWER THE QUESTIONS.**

1. The nurse should ascertain exactly when and where Chelsea and her father were camping, and if either remembers a tick bite. The incidence for most tick-borne infections is highest in the spring and summer. Additionally, most ticks live in grasses and plants, especially in heavily wooded areas. Timing is also important to determine the stage of the disease. For example, the early, localized stage occurs 3 to 30 days after the tick bite. Treatment during the early stage helps to prevent other manifestations, including later stages of the disease. The nurse also needs to assess for other signs and symptoms, such as fever, chills, malaise, and evidence of other areas of rash that appear smaller than the original area.

2. The treatment for Lyme disease erythema migrans and early disease is doxycycline. This drug is given to children older than 8 years; if Chelsea was younger than 8 years of age, amoxicillin would be used. If she was allergic to penicillin, she most likely would receive cefuroxime, because she is younger than 9 years of age. Chelsea would receive treatment for 14 to 21 days. If Chelsea had early disseminated disease or late Lyme disease, she would receive intravenous penicillin or ceftriaxone for 14 to 28 days.

3. Prevention is a key aspect of teaching for Chelsea and her parents. They need instruction on how to avoid tick attachment, such as spraying clothing with tick repellant; wearing light colors and long sleeves, long pants, shoes, and socks; and checking the skin frequently when outdoors. They also need teaching on how to remove ticks safely Although Chelsea is not contagious, the parents should notify the school nurse that Chelsea is being treated to help dispel unwarranted fear among her classmates.

SECTION III: PRACTICING FOR NCLEX

Activity D **CHOOSE THE BEST ANSWER.**

1. c   **2.** d   **3.** b   **4.** d   **5.** a
6. b   **7.** c

CHAPTER 25

SECTION I: ASSESSING YOUR UNDERSTANDING

Activity A **FILL IN THE BLANKS.**

1. Melanin
2. Eosinophils
3. Seborrheic dermatitis
4. Fomites

5. Group A beta-hemolytic streptococcal (GABHS) and *Staphylococcus aureus*
6. Virus
7. Fungal infections
8. Pressure ulcers
9. Urushiol
10. Angioedema

Activity B **MATCH THE TYPES OF DERMATITIS IN COLUMN A WITH THEIR CAUSE IN COLUMN B.**

1. c   **2.** d   **3.** b   **4.** a

Activity C **WRITE THE CORRECT SEQUENCE IN THE BOXES PROVIDED.**

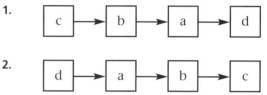

1. c → b → a → d

2. d → a → b → c

Activity D **BRIEFLY ANSWER THE FOLLOWING.**

1. Treatment intervention for candidiasis involves three primary interventions:

   a. Removal of any predisposing cause or use of a preventive petroleum, zinc oxide, or dimethicone water-repellent ointment to prevent the causative agent from continually reinfecting the area may be required if inflammation is severe.

   b. Apply topical or oral antifungal agents such as nystatin, miconazole, clotrimazole, and ketoconazole. Improvement should be noted within 3 to 5 days.

   c. Keep the affected area dry.

2. There are four stages of skin ulcers. In stage I, the pressure ulcer is an observable pressure-related alteration of intact skin with indicators, compared with an adjacent or opposite area on the body, that may include changes in one or more of the following: skin temperature (warmth or coolness), tissue consistency (firm or boggy feel), and/or sensation (pain, itching). The ulcer appears as a defined area of persistent redness in lightly pigmented skin, whereas in darker skin tones, the ulcer may appear with persistent red, blue, or purple hues. Stage II involves partial-thickness skin loss of epidermis or dermis. The ulcer is superficial and presents clinically as an abrasion, a blister, or a shallow crater. Stage III is represented by full-thickness skin loss involving damage to or necrosis of subcutaneous tissue that may extend down to, but not through, underlying fascia. The ulcer presents clinically as a deep crater with or without undermining of adjacent tissue. Stage IV is full-thickness skin loss with extensive destruction, tissue necrosis, or damage to

muscle, bone, or supporting structures (e.g., tendon or joint capsule). Undermining and sinus tracts may also be associated with stage IV pressure ulcers.

SECTION II: APPLYING YOUR KNOWLEDGE

Activity E CONSIDER THE SCENARIO AND ANSWER THE QUESTIONS.

1. Jordan has sustained burns on approximately 38% of his body.
2. The following are appropriate nursing diagnoses for a burn patient:
   a. Ineffective airway clearance related to upper airway edema
   b. Risk for infection related to broken skin barrier
   c. Pain related to injured skin
   d. Altered tissue perfusion related to hypovolemia
   e. Disturbed body image related to altered body appearance.
3. Answers:
   a. Fluid and Electrolyte Deficits: In addition to the large amount of intravascular fluid volume lost during burn shock, a child has a larger body mass-to-surface area ratio than an adult, thus increasing the extent of heat and evaporative water loss.
   b. Hypermetabolism characterizes the metabolic response to burn injury and occurs in proportion to the extent of the burn. Energy expenditures may increase from 40% to 100% above basal levels in children with burns of more than 30% TBSA. Core body temperature for a child with a major burn injury will reset at about 99.5 to 100.4 °F (37.5–38 °C), or 99 °F, and will remain at that level or higher until skin coverage is achieved.
   c. Hyperglycemia is common after burn injury, because glucose metabolism is also altered.
   d. Infection: The warm moist environment of a major burn wound is an ideal location for bacterial growth. Wound infection is a great risk, because a burn injury presents a source of organisms capable of producing disease, a mode of transmission, and a susceptible host.

SECTION III: PRACTICING FOR NCLEX

Activity F CHOOSE THE BEST ANSWER.

1. **Answer: b**
   RATIONALE: Mongolian spots are blue-black macules or patches commonly located on the lumbosacral area. They are most common in Asian, black, and Hispanic infants. The sacrococcygeal area is most commonly affected, but lesions may occur on the buttocks, dorsal trunk, or extremities. Mongolian spots generally fade by age 2 to 3 years, although some traces of the lesions may persist into adulthood.

2. **Answer: a**
   RATIONALE: Cultures of the lesions from erythema toxicum neonatorium (ETN) are sterile. A crucial factor differentiating ETN from other skin disorders is that, aside from eruption of the lesions, the neonate displays no other systemic involvement such as fever, lethargy, or poor feeding.

3. **Answer: d**
   RATIONALE: The goals of therapy include rehydrating the skin, removing scales, preventing infection, inhibiting the pathologic process and suppressing the immune response, and promoting acceptance of the child's condition. Complete recovery is rare. Psoriasis is not contagious, so contact with other children is not necessary.

4. **Answer: b**
   RATIONALE: Oral antibiotics are the most common systemic therapy prescribed for acne vulgaris. Daily oral medications should be taken at the same time each day to increase effectiveness. Abrasive soaps and astringents should not be used, because these products only serve to cause drying and peeling of the skin, and fail to prevent the lesions from appearing. Specific food restrictions have not been shown to be beneficial in the treatment of acne. Advise the adolescent not to "pop" pimples, because doing so can cause further inflammation at the site and scarring at sites of larger lesions.

5. **Answer: b**
   RATIONALE: Instruct parents to follow the prescribed treatment plan carefully. Improper application of over-the-counter treatments that contain lindane can lead to toxic side effects. These may include nausea, vomiting, aplastic anemia, hypoplastic bone marrow, convulsions, and death. Pets are not a host for lice. When teaching parents about pediculicide treatment, emphasize that more is not better. Directions for application must be strictly followed.

6. **Answer: a**
   RATIONALE: HPV is transmitted predominantly through sexual contact. Warts of the genitalia in young children should raise the question of possible sexual abuse. Daily hygiene does not affect the presence of warts. Undergarments have no bearing on the spread or manifestation of HPV. Assessment of home treatments is a good idea, but not more important than assessment for sexual abuse.

7. **Answer: c**
   RATIONALE: Fungal skin infections can be life-threatening when the child is nutritionally depleted or is immunocompromised. Assessment of daily hygiene is important, but not as vital as the nutrition assessment. Fungal skin infections do not involve the respiratory tract. There are no current immunizations for fungal skin infections.

8. **Answer: b**
   RATIONALE: The lesion sites of a fungal skin infection should be cleansed thoroughly with water

before applying any medications. Students participating in athletics should be encouraged to change
their socks and shoes immediately after a sports
activity and to expose their feet to warm, dry air
by wearing sandals or thongs. Children with tinea
infections should refrain from applying oils or
petroleum jelly to their skin or scalp because these
agents act as an occlusive medium and can promote more fungal growth. Removal of scales is not
necessary.

9. **Answer: c**
RATIONALE: Prevention of pressure ulcers is the best
nursing care. The remainder of these answers are
correct nursing care for pressure ulcers, however
the best care is always prevention.

10. **Answer: a**
RATIONALE: Each of the interventions are appropriate, however the most immediate action would be
to stop the suspected drug.

11. **Answer: c**
RATIONALE: Carbon monoxide inhalation and
hypoxia are treated by administering high concentrations of oxygen by mask until the condition is
resolved. The semi–Fowler's position is not necessary, intubation may not be necessary, and placing
an oxygen saturation probe is not the first priority.

12. **Answer: d**
RATIONALE: The mother is most likely correct. The
most common presenting symptom of scabies is
pruritus, which is especially profound at night and
at nap time. An itchy scalp could also be a symptom of head lice. Transmission of scabies can be
through fomites as well as through close contact
with an infected person.

13. **Answer: c**
RATIONALE: Hand, foot, and mouth disease is highly
contagious and almost impossible to prevent its
spread. It is highly likely the older sibling will catch
it. Humans are the only known hosts, so avoiding
pets is not necessary. The child can return to daycare as soon as her fever is gone for 24 hours.

14. **Answer: a**
RATIONALE: Taking a shower directly after contact
with other wrestlers and contaminated mats will
help prevent the spread of ringworm. Dogs can be
carriers of ringworm. A person can be a carrier of
ringworm even if lesions are not visible. Medication should be taken until completed to prevent
reinfection.

15. **Answer: a**
RATIONALE: Daily saline baths are a primary supportive intervention, along with applying antibiotic ointments to the eroded areas and antibiotic
mesh gauze to denuded areas. The use of silver sul-
fadiazine cream and the liberal use of viscous lidocaine is contraindicated.

16. **Answer: c**
RATIONALE: Dressing changes for burns should be
performed as quickly as possible to minimize pain.

Removing a parent from the room could upset the
child. The parents may stay for the procedure if
they wish. Giving an oral medication just before
the procedure does not give it enough time to be
absorbed and take effect. Painful procedures
should be done in a treatment room if possible to
maintain the child's room as a safe place.

17. **Answer: b**
RATIONALE: Regression to a former developmental
level is not uncommon during a hospital stay.
Reassuring the child that diaper use is acceptable
behavior is the most appropriate action for the
nurse to take. Reminding a child of past behaviors
and implying that a child is no longer a "big girl"
is not effective or supportive nursing actions.

18. **Answer: d**
RATIONALE: Short-term memory loss is important
for the parents to understand right away. Using
technical terms such as *myoglobinuria* to explain
conditions that may or may not happen is not
helpful. Pointing out wounds that the parents can
already see is not beneficial. Arrhythmias are associated with electrical injuries, however they occur
immediately after the event and would have been
already resolved.

CHAPTER 26

SECTION I: ASSESSING YOUR UNDERSTANDING

Activity A MATCH THE DESCRIPTION IN
COLUMN A WITH THE APPROPRIATE ANSWER
IN COLUMN B.

1. b   **2.** e   **3.** d   **4.** a   **5.** c

Activity B MATCH THE ALTERED ENDOCRINE
FUNCTION IN COLUMN A WITH THE CORRECT
DEFINITION IN COLUMN B.

1. d   **2.** a   **3.** e   **4.** b   **5.** c

Activity C PLACE THE FOLLOWING STEPS OF
NEGATIVE FEEDBACK IN THEIR PROPER
SEQUENCE.

1.
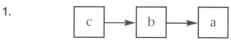

Activity D FILL IN THE BLANKS.

1. Panhypopituitarism
2. Congenital hypothyroidism
3. Thyrotoxicosis
4. Hyperparathyroidism
5. Diabetes

SECTION II: APPLYING YOUR KNOWLEDGE

Activity E BRIEFLY ANSWER THE FOLLOWING.

1. Type 2 diabetes is most often associated with obesity, hypertension, and elevated cholesterol (combined hyperlipidemia). The condition may also be associated with metabolic syndrome. It is also associated with acromegaly, Cushing's Syndrome, and a number of other endocrinologic disorders, including polycystic ovarian syndrome (PCOS).

2. It has been hypothesized that an environmental trigger initiates the autoimmune process that ultimately results in progressive dysfunction of the adrenal gland and the subsequent adrenal insufficiency of Addison's disease, but no such trigger has yet been defined. Risk for adrenal autoimmunity is considered genetic. Many relatives of individuals with Addison's disease have other autoimmune diseases, such as type 1 diabetes or autoimmune thyroid disease.

3. Prolonged hypersecretion results in adrenal gland hyperplasia and sex steroid overproduction. In females, this condition causes masculinization or virilization of the clitoris. In males, it may cause precocious puberty. Children with CAH who cannot maintain a sodium balance [salt-losing form of Congenital Adrenal Hyperplasia (CAH)], if they are not diagnosed and treated promptly, are at increased risk for severe hyponatremic dehydration, seizures, shock, and death from this electrolyte imbalance.

Activity F CONSIDER THE SCENARIO AND ANSWER THE QUESTIONS.

1. Type 1 diabetes has no single cause, although certain common characteristics can precede diagnosis, including seasonal variations (midwinter and spring) and a history of illness, emotional stress, or infection immediately preceding diagnosis. Many patients with type 1 diabetes have no prior affected family member. The incidence of type 1 diabetes in children increases with age throughout childhood and reaches its peak at puberty.

2. Insulin deficiency and resistance cause physiologic and metabolic changes throughout the body. Because of the insulin deficiency, glucose derived from dietary sources cannot be used by the cells (specifically muscle and fat cells) and begins to increase in the bloodstream (hyperglycemia).

3. Long-term complications such as disorders of the eye (diabetic retinopathy), kidney (diabetic nephropathy), circulatory system (heart disease, stroke), and nerve fibers (peripheral neuropathy) are common secondary conditions associated with diabetes. If left untreated, type 1 diabetes can result in death.

SECTION III: PRACTICING FOR NCLEX

Activity G CHOOSE THE BEST ANSWER.

1. **Answer: b**
   RATIONALE: This medication is given to treat hypothyroidism. Increased doses of Synthroid can produce signs and symptoms of hyperthyroidism, such as tachycardia, angina, tremors, nervousness, insomnia, hyperthermia, heat intolerance, and sweating. The patient should call the doctor if these occur.

2. **Answer: c**
   RATIONALE: Roughly 60% of the mass of the body is water, and despite wide variation in the amount of water taken in each day, body water content remains incredibly stable. Such precise control of body water and solute concentrations is a function of several hormones acting on both the kidneys and the vascular system. Antidiuretic hormone (vasopressin) is very important in this process and should be monitored by the nurse.

3. **Answer: c**
   RATIONALE: Glucagon has a major role in maintaining normal concentrations of glucose in blood and is often described as having the opposite effect of insulin. That is, glucagon has the effect of increasing blood glucose levels. The major effect of glucagon is to stimulate an increase in blood concentration of glucose.

4. **Answer: d**
   RATIONALE: Calcium is what the nervous system of our body uses to conduct electricity. This is why the most common symptoms of parathyroid disease and high calcium levels are related to nervous system issues such as depression, weakness, and tiredness. When the calcium levels are not correct, people can feel weak and have muscle cramps.

5. **Answer: c**
   RATIONALE: Many menstrual problems may be symptoms of undiagnosed thyroid conditions. Girls who have either very early or very late menstruation should be evaluated for a potential thyroid problem, because thyroid problems can frequently be a cause of early or delayed puberty and menstruation. Hyperthyroidism in a teenage girl can delay the onset of puberty and onset of menstruation into the mid teens, in some cases after the age of 15.

6. **Answer: c**
   RATIONALE: Hyperthyroidism occurs less often in children than hypothyroidism. Graves' disease, the most common cause of hyperthyroidism in children, occurs in 1 in 5,000 children between 11 and 15 years of age. Hyperthyroidism occurs more often in females, and the peak incidence occurs during adolescence.

7. **Answer: c**
   RATIONALE: Diagnosis is based on a positive history of the signs and symptoms of hypoparathyroidism, and on the physical examination. Assess for the presence of positive Chvostek or Trousseau signs, both of which indicate hypocalcemia.

8. **Answer: a**
   RATIONALE: Strong family history of type 2 is often present, as is a familial tendency toward obesity and a sedentary lifestyle. A child whose mother had gestational diabetes is particularly at risk for diabetes. Although ethnic background and the mother's gestational history are not a modifiable risk factor, weight and lifestyle certainly are.

9. **Answer: b**
   RATIONALE: Chronic adrenocortical insufficiency (Addison's disease) is commonly caused by autoimmune destruction of the adrenal cortex, which results in dysfunction of steroidogenesis. The condition usually occurs during early adolescence. Addison's disease has become more common in children through its association with type 1 diabetes. Patients with type 1 diabetes are at increased risk for Addison's disease: Approximately 1% of patients with this type of diabetes have the autoantibodies associated with Addison's disease.

10. **Answer: c**
    RATIONALE: The more common cause of Cushing's Syndrome in children is side effects of prolonged or excessive treatment with exogenous corticosteroids for a medical condition such as asthma, lupus, or inflammatory bowel disease. Most of these side effects can be reversed once the corticosteroid treatment is reduced or the doses are gradually tapered. Excess cortisol produces diverse side effects seen throughout the body. The most noticeable side effect is obesity or rapid weight gain with arrest in linear growth.

CHAPTER 27

SECTION I: ASSESSING YOUR UNDERSTANDING

Activity A FILL IN THE BLANKS.
1. Metabolizing
2. Newborn screening
3. Early recognition
4. Phenylketonuria
5. Recessive

Activity B MATCH THE TERMS RELATED TO METABOLIC DISORDERS LISTED IN COLUMN A WITH THEIR DEFINITIONS LISTED IN COLUMN B.
1. e   2. b   3. a   4. d   5. c
6. f

Activity C BRIEFLY ANSWER THE FOLLOWING.
1. A crisis can develop rapidly in the presence of a metabolic disturbance and can cause irreversible symptoms or death. Therefore, identifying the cause of symptoms accurately and quickly is essential. A thorough physical assessment should be completed by the physician or advance practice nurse.

2. Abnormalities commonly revealed during a physical examination focused on neurodevelopmental functions include impaired states of alertness and arousal, tremors, posturing, clonic jerking, tonic spasms, or seizures.

3. Generally, disorders included in screening programs are those with relatively high prevalence, clinical symptoms that are not present until irreversible damage occurs, clinical manifestations severe enough to make an impact on society, treatments that are known and facilities available to provide treatment, diagnostic evaluation possible through a simple method of collection, and follow-up available if test results are abnormal.

4. High-pressure gas–liquid chromatography, ion exchange chromatography, mass spectroscopy, and electron microscopy are used to analyze blood, plasma, urine, or cerebrospinal fluid to detect metabolic disorders.

5. A healthcare team should consider and suspect a metabolic disorder when a neonate becomes severely ill, when developmental milestones are not met, or when developmental regression begins to appear in the previously healthy child.

6. Treatment interventions include decreasing substrates preceding the enzymatic block, administering a supplement of the deficient product that should have been produced, providing an enzymatic cofactor, using medications to remove accumulated substrates, replacing deficient enzymes through intravenous administration, undergoing liver or bone marrow transplantation to eliminate all deficient enzymes, and providing somatic gene therapy (future option).

Activity D MATCH THE DEFINITIONS IN COLUMN A WITH THE DISORDERS LISTED IN COLUMN B.
1. b   2. d   3. c   4. e   5. a

Activity E CONSIDER THE SCENARIO AND ANSWER THE QUESTIONS.
1. Initial signs of maple syrup urine disease (MSUD) include poor feeding, a maple syrup odor in cerumen, ketonuria, and vomiting, which occur within 48 hours of delivery. The Guthrie test is slow. By the time Guthrie results are available, MSUD could already have been detected through other methods and a clinical examination. If a suspicion of MSUD exists, testing done routinely includes plasma

amino acids and urine organic acids. Ketonuria as detected by use of standard urine strip tests is present in MSUD. Additional laboratory findings that indicate MSUD are increased levels of leucine, isoleucine, valine, keto acids, and alloisoleucine in both plasma and urine.

2. The management goals for MSUD are to establish an early diagnosis, to remove the toxic metabolites, and to prevent tissue catabolism. Long-term treatment includes dietary leucine restriction, high-calorie BCAA-free formulas, and frequent monitoring. Liver transplantation is a reasonable treatment option for classic MSUD (Strauss, Puffenberger & Morton, 2006).

3. The family may feel frightened by the changes in their child's condition and the need to be moved to the intensive care unit. The nurse should work with the social worker and child life specialist to provide support and teaching to assist the family through the crisis associated with the initial diagnosis and rigorous treatment methods.

SECTION III: PRACTICING FOR NCLEX

Activity F CHOOSE THE BEST ANSWER.

1. **Answer: c**
   RATIONALE: Tay-Sachs disease, Gaucher's disease, and Niemann-Pick disease occur more frequently among individuals of Ashkenazi Jewish descent. Phenylketonuria is most common among Jews of Yemenite origin The tyrosine defect tyrosinemia type I has a higher prevalence in patients with a French Canadian ancestry. The classic form of maple syrup urine disease is more common among members of Mennonite and Amish sects.

2. **Answer: b**
   RATIONALE: A musty, mousy smell is associated with PKU. Hypermethioninemia has a boiled cabbage, rancid butter smell, Multiple carboxylase deficiency has a cat urine smell as an indicator. A symptom of hawkinsinuria is a distinctive swimming pool smell.

3. **Answer: a**
   RATIONALE: Hemochromatosis is an accumulation of iron that can cause extensive tissue damage if not treated. Acrodermatitis enteropathica is a systemic zinc deficiency. Primary hypomagnesemia is an intestinal malabsorption of magnesium, and Fabry's disease is a deficiency of alpha-galactosidase.

4. **Answer: d**
   RATIONALE: Gaucher's disease is caused by deficient beta-glucosidase. Neiman-Pick disease is caused by deficient sphingomyelinase, Tay-Sachs disease is caused by deficient hexosaminidase A, and Hunter's disease is caused by deficient iduronate sulfatase.

5. **Answer: a**
   RATIONALE: Elevations in BUN and creatinine indicate renal involvement, as seen in conditions such as Wilson's disease.

6. **Answer: b**
   RATIONALE: Mitochondrial disease will show alterations in muscle tissue.

7. **Answer: c**
   RATIONALE: Foods low in copper include beef, eggs, turkey and chicken (white meat only), cold cuts containing no pork, organ meats or dark meat, most vegetables except mushrooms and avocados, most fruits, and refined flour products.

8. **Answer: d**
   RATIONALE: The following metabolic conditions occur during the neonatal period: galactosemia, hyperammonemia, hyperglycinemia, isovaleric acidemia, maple syrup disease, Menkes disease, phenylketonuria, sulfite oxidase deficiency, and tyrosinemia type I (acute form).

9. **Answer: a**
   RATIONALE: The nurse should make sure Jonnie understands her diet and can explain it to friends who ask questions about it. The parents should allow Jonnie to determine when to eat the medical food. Genetic and pregnancy counseling should be provided to adolescents with PKU.

10. **Answer: d**
    RATIONALE: All newborns should complete newborn screening before discharge from the newborn nursery, preferably between 24 and 72 hours of age, and in no case later than 7 days of life. Screening should be completed before transfusion or dialysis.

Activity G CHOOSE ALL ANSWERS THAT APPLY.

1. **Answer: b, c, d**
   RATIONALE: Common to most metabolic problems is a history of poor feeding, including rejection or dislike of protein foods, vomiting, listlessness, failure to thrive, delayed development, and increasing weakness.

2. **Answer: b, c, d, e**
   RATIONALE: The significant clinical features of tyrosinemia type I are poor appetite and failure to grow normally, vomiting, diarrhea, bloody stools, a cabbagelike odor, jaundice, swollen liver, irritability, lethargy, liver cirrhosis, and kidney problems.

Activity H FILL IN THE BLANKS.

1. Medical foods
2. Gene therapy
3. Phenylketonuria

CHAPTER 28

SECTION I: ASSESSING YOUR UNDERSTANDING

Activity A MATCH THE ALTERATION IN VISION IN COLUMN A WITH THE PROPER PHRASE OR TERM IN COLUMN B.

1. b   **2.** a   **3.** e   **4.** f   **5.** c
6. d

Activity B MATCH THE ALTERATION IN HEARING IN COLUMN A WITH PHRASE OR TERM IN COLUMN B.

1. c   **2.** e   **3.** b   **4.** d   **5.** a

Activity C PLACE THE FOLLOWING DEVELOPMENTAL STAGES FOR VISION IN THE PROPER ORDER.

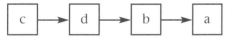

Activity D FILL IN THE BLANKS.

1. accurate
2. intensity
3. cooperate
4. glaucoma
5. conjunctivitis
6. intensity and pitch
7. spoken communication
8. Hoarseness

SECTION II: APPLYING YOUR KNOWLEDGE

Activity E BRIEFLY ANSWER THE FOLLOWING.

1. The four ways in which nurses facilitate screening and prevention of vision, hearing, and communication disorders are as follows: promoting early identification and treatment of sensory alterations, assisting and teaching parents and children how to prevent or minimize trauma that could affect sensory abilities, helping parents to find ways to promote the development of the permanently impaired child, and developing and implementing a care plan for the child with altered sensory function.
2. A speech disorder includes impairment in articulation of speech sounds, fluency, or voice. A child with a speech disorder may have difficulty saying certain sounds after the time when he or she should have developmentally learned those sounds, or may stutter after the time when brief repetitions or pauses are normal. Language disorders are of two different types: receptive language disorders and expressive language disorders. Receptive language disorders include impairment in comprehension; expressive language disorders affect the use of language in verbal, written, or symbol form. The child with a language disorder may be unable to understand what is being said to them or may have difficulty responding appropriately.
3. Conductive hearing loss occurs when sound is prevented from reaching the auditory nerve. Sound intensity is insufficient to allow hearing. Therefore, a hearing aid that amplifies sound is an effective intervention. Sensorineural hearing loss exists when the cochlea does not relay sound pattern information received from the middle ear. Hearing is affected not only in terms of intensity, but also in terms of pitch. Cochlear implants convert sound into electrical signals and transmit them to the auditory nerve.
4. The loss of both hearing and sight may be a result of a congenital defect, acquired illness, or injury. In many cases, the loss of hearing and vision can affect the child's spoken communication. Vision and hearing deficits are seldom complete. It is important to identify the child's residual abilities and they must be used to maximal benefit. The desired outcome for a child that has multiple sensory challenges is for them to have the opportunity to develop to their maximal potential.

Activity F CONSIDER THE SCENARIO AND ANSWER THE QUESTIONS.

1. As the nurse, you should observe external ocular structures, looking for size, shape, and symmetry of the eyes, as well as the lashes, eyebrows, and other structures of the eye. Note any ptosis, slanting, or deviation from normal findings. John's ocular motility should also be assessed. Instruct John to follow an object such as a colorful pencil. His eyes should move symmetrically and remain fixed on the object, and both eyes should work together. Allow the toy or testing object to pause at each of the six positions. The normal response is for both eyes to follow the test object to each of the six cardinal positions of gaze. If an eye muscle is weak, the eye may be unable to reach the position or may not hold it. The child's response may be to blink and abandon the position with the stronger eye as well. The cover/uncover test may also be used. Visual acuity should be assessed using a Snellen chart or equivalent. Visual acuity for John's age should be 20/30 or 20/20. An assessment of John's visual fields is also important. By age 3 years, most children can cooperate with the examiner sufficiently for a full visual assessment, which includes assessment of visual fields. Have the child cover one eye and look at your nose. Hold your finger out to the side at arm's length and equidistant between you and the child's eyes. Wiggle your finger and move it in from the periphery. Ask the child to say

"now" when he or she can first see it without moving his or her head or eyes. Test each eye separately and compare the amplitude of the child's field of vision with your own. If you identify a diminished visual field, a full funduscopic examination must be completed immediately and the child should be referred to an eye care specialist.

2. Know the treatment protocol being used, and your responsibility in assisting the child and family to follow it. Learn the appropriate patching technique. As the nurse, you may be responsible for changing the patch should it become loose and/or soiled. The school should have a copy of the written treatment plan on file. As the school nurse, you should provide education to John's class about his special eye patch so the children understand. The teacher and daycare providers may need to discourage teasing and educate the other children concerning the reason the child wears the eye patch. Other children can learn to be helpful in the treatment program and continued social development of the individual child.

3. Amblyopia, if detected early, is treatable. The earlier the condition is identified and treatment is begun, the greater the likelihood of a positive outcome. Because development at young ages is more rapid, improvement may occur more quickly if the child is younger when treatment begins, and the best time to treat children with amblyopia is when they are younger than 7 years of age. Compliance with the treatment regime is vital. If warranted, surgery and medications are additional treatment modalities.

SECTION III: PRACTICING FOR NCLEX
Activity G CHOOSE THE BEST ANSWER.

1. **Answer: a**
   RATIONALE: A playmate with pink eye would provide an excellent opportunity for infection. Allergic reaction to dust mites would not cause infectious conjunctivitis. Recent cerumen impaction and a family history of conjunctivitis are not contributing factors for infectious conjunctivitis.

2. **Answer: b**
   RATIONALE: Lack of interest in feeding and increased irritability are signs of a generalized response to the infective agent. Edema of the eyelids is typical of older infants and children who can rub their eyes. Inflammation and purulent discharge are initial symptoms of the disorder.

3. **Answer: c**
   RATIONALE: A blue tinge to the sclera may be a sign of glaucoma in a newborn. A white, opaque appearance of the lens and absence of the red reflex are indications of cataracts. Copious purulent drainage is a sign of ophthalmia neonatorum.

4. **Answer: d**
   RATIONALE: Myopia results from excessive refractive power being exerted on the lens. The light rays are focused in front of the retina rather than on the retina. Anisometropia occurs when both eyes have refractive errors, and the errors are considerably different. Hyperopia results from either a short axial length or decreased curvature of the lens. In astigmatism, the shape and curvature of the cornea are not symmetric; thus, light rays are not focused symmetrically.

5. **Answer: d**
   RATIONALE: The classic sign of acute otitis media is pain on movement of the pinna or pain on pressure over the tragus. Symptoms of upper respiratory infection many times accompany otitis media, but do not affect otitis externa. The tympanic membrane reacting to a puff of air is a sign that there is no fluid buildup in the middle ear. The absence of cerumen in the ear canal is not a symptom of otitis externa.

6. **Answer: c**
   RATIONALE: The incidence of amblyopia may be higher than usual among some groups of children, such as those born of drug-dependent mothers. Chemical conjunctivitis is caused by antibiotic prophylaxis and is not related to amblyopia. A mild eye injury would not result in amblyopia. Frequent upper respiratory infections contribute to otitis media, not amblyopia.

7. **Answer: d**
   RATIONALE: Usually, the ear infection appears a few days after the onset of an upper respiratory infection. Organisms gain entrance to the middle ear through the eustachian tube. Tobacco smoke exposure does play a role in the development of otitis media. Children's eustachian tubes are shorter, wider, and more horizontal than adults. The high incidence in infants and young children of otitis media does not decrease until 9 years of age.

8. **Answer: b**
   RATIONALE: The entire family needs to learn good hand washing techniques because they are key to preventing infection within the family. Directing the parents to use a full course of medication is very important to help prevent a recurrence in the child. Telling of a possible cause has little preventative value, as does proper administration of medication.

9. **Answer: c**
   RATIONALE: The absence of the red reflex and a white, opaque appearance of the lens are tell-tale signs of a cataract. Ptosis of the eye lids could be a result of the injury, but not a sign of cataracts. Itchy eyes is a sign of eye irritation. Edema of the eyelids is a sign of allergic conjunctivitis.

10. **Answer: d**
    RATIONALE: Silver nitrate 1% is an antibacterial prophylaxis that may cause conjunctivitis. Retinopathy of prematurity is an overgrowth of retinal blood vessels. Cataracts may be caused by genetics or may be acquired after birth. The inability of the aqueous humor to drain from the eye is a result of glaucoma.

CHAPTER 29

SECTION I: ASSESSING YOUR UNDERSTANDING

Activity A **MATCH THE KEY TERM IN COLUMN A WITH THE CORRECT DEFINITION IN COLUMN B.**

1. b   **2.** a   **3.** d   **4.** e   **5.** c

Activity B **MATCH THE PSYCHOTROPIC MEDICATION CLASSIFICATION IN COLUMN A WITH AN EXAMPLE OF THIS MEDICATION IN COLUMN B.**

1. d   **2.** i   **3.** g   **4.** e   **5.** c
6. f   **7.** b   **8.** j   **9.** h   **10.** a

Activity C **PLACE THE FOLLOWING STEPS IN THE COGNITIVE BEHAVIOR THERAPEUTIC PROCESS IN THE PROPER ORDER.**

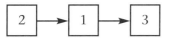

Activity D **FILL IN THE BLANKS.**

1. Suicide
2. Dysthymia
3. Somatic
4. 4
5. Thermometers
6. Conduct
7. Serotonin
8. 10
9. Cognitive–behavioral
10. Bipolar disorder

Activity E **NAME EACH OF THE FIVE AXES OF THE DSM-IV DIAGNOSTIC CLASSIFICATIONS.**

Axis i: Clinical disorders, other conditions that are focus of clinical attention
Axis ii: Personality disorders, mental retardation
Axis iii: General medical conditions
Axis iv: Psychosocial, environmental problems
Axis v: Global assessment of functioning

SECTION II: APPLYING YOUR KNOWLEDGE

Activity F **BRIEFLY ANSWER THE QUESTIONS.**

1. No, they are two different terms. Delinquency implies committing criminal or illegal acts; it is a legal term. Conduct disorder is a diagnostic term.
2. It is a pattern of negative, resistant, and hostile behavior that usually manifests after early childhood and before puberty.
3. A common way to for adolescents to communicate about suicidal thoughts is through a friend. Examples: They may talk about "a friend" who is considering suicide when they are indirectly talking about their own concerns. They may pass a note or ask a classmate about committing suicide. They may make the threat of suicide to a friend.
4. Substance abuse is defined as a pattern of continued and inappropriate use of substances that causes substantial emotional, psychological, and physiologic effects.

Activity G **CONSIDER THE SCENARIO AND ANSWER THE QUESTIONS.**

1. The mental status examination focuses on behavioral observations made of the child or adolescent's appearance and behavior during 2 to 3 hours of interview. With children and adolescents, the mental status examination also includes information from parents and teachers about how the child interacts with peers.
2. Evaluate children with oppositional defiant disorder (ODD) for depression. The underlying problem may be continuous unmanageable life stresses and multiple losses. Dysthymia or depressive traits may mimic ODD. ODD is also strongly associated with anxiety disorders. Mismanagement and lack of recognition of these underlying problems may lead to ODD.
3. Potential outcomes for children with ODD vary. In many cases, without early and effective treatment, Conduct Disorder (CD) and even criminal behavior ensue, resulting in incarceration. Other less severe problems are academic difficulties or failure, and continuous peer conflict, which may result in injury.

SECTION III: PRACTICING FOR THE NCLEX

Activity H **CHOOSE THE BEST ANSWER.**

1. **Answer: d**
   RATIONALE: Reassurance along with a concrete solution such as attending a local support group comprised of other parents of schizophrenic children is the best immediate response in this situation. Information about the illness and its onset would do little to reassure them. Telling them that an accurate diagnosis can take several years might give them false hopes. Telling them to be strong is not helpful.
2. **Answer: d**
   RATIONALE: Asking the girl an open-ended question about her sore throat could open a dialogue for the nurse to bring up her concerns regarding bulimia in a nonthreatening way. Asking the girl to step on the scale might put the girl on the defensive, because patients suffering from eating disorders are hypersensitive about their weight. Directly mentioning bulimia and pointing out the damage to the girl's teeth might also be received defensively.
3. **Answer: a**
   RATIONALE: The most immediate goal of the nurse is to reduce anxiety to a manageable level and to

reduce the child's physical discomfort. Encouraging the child both to breathe deeply and to focus on a comforting object or thought is an immediate action the child can take to achieve the primary goal. The nurse should call the child's parents and try to determine what preceded the attack.

4. **Answer: b**
   RATIONALE: Because the nurse suspects separation anxiety, the best approach is to involve both the child and parent. This statement also subtly engages and validates the mother as a member of the team helping her daughter. Telling the mother her daughter might have separation anxiety could further upset the mother. Letting the mother vent her frustration might be helpful to the mother, but it will be nonproductive. Asking the mother her opinion will provide helpful information, but the nurse's first goal is to encourage the mother to calm down and enlist her assistance.

5. **Answer: a**
   RATIONALE: Teaching the child relaxation techniques empowers her to counter stressful feelings on her own. A daily exercise program is also important, but mentioning the child's physical education class might bring up a source of stress. It is best to work with the parents to ensure regular exercise. Positive affirmations are helpful, but less appropriate in this case because of the girl's age. Implying that the girl is partially to blame for her stress is not helpful.

6. **Answer: a**
   RATIONALE: The nurse must first make sure that the parents understand that many children with anxiety disorders do not respond to medication. When the parents understand the facts about medication, the nurse should then emphasize the importance of the family understanding the anxiety disorder as well as the key role of therapy in the treatment plan. Finally, the nurse should make sure that the parents are comfortable with their son's treatment plan and develop a shared definition for improvement.

7. **Answer: b**
   RATIONALE: The first action would be to implement crisis intervention to help the child through the initial trauma and to educate the family to facilitate the child's recovery. Informing the child that her mother passed away is inappropriate. Contacting the girl's teachers is not the first priority. Scheduling a session with a cognitive therapist will be helpful, but again, this is not the first priority.

8. **Answer: c**
   RATIONALE: This question is nonthreatening and open ended. It addresses the specific issue of the child's perception of her body image in appropriate language. "Do you think you look healthy?" and "Do you like what you see?" would most likely elicit yes or no answers. "Did you know that you could suffer permanent damage?" could be perceived as threatening and is not helpful.

9. **Answer: c**
   RATIONALE: Remind the parents that they must have reasonable expectations. The problem developed over many months and will not be resolved in a week. Keeping a night light on and leaving the door open are appropriate interventions, but do not address the parents' impatience. Advising them to avoid excessive anger and abusive discipline is unnecessary, and the parents might take offense.

10. **Answer: b**
    RATIONALE: The nurse's goal is to clearly explain the rules and firmly yet empathically adhere to them. The nurse shows no empathy when she says she does not make the rules. Telling the boy that she is concerned he might hurt himself does not address the rules and could possibly further upset him by drawing attention to his previous injuries. Letting the boy keep the pencil violates the rules.

CHAPTER 30

SECTION I: ASSESSING YOUR UNDERSTANDING

Activity A MATCH THE TEST NAME IN COLUMN A WITH THE PROPER PHRASE IN COLUMN B.

1. e   **2.** a   **3.** b   **4.** c   **5.** d

Activity B MATCH THE DIAGNOSTIC MODALITY IN COLUMN A WITH THE CORRECT PHRASE IN COLUMN B.

1. b   **2.** e   **3.** a   **4.** d   **5.** c

Activity C FILL IN THE BLANKS.

1. Strengths
2. Intelligence
3. Functional
4. Advocate
5. Empathy
6. Nurturing and stimulation
7. History
8. Milestone
9. Adaptive
10. Failure and frustration

SECTION II: APPLYING YOUR KNOWLEDGE

Activity D BRIEFLY ANSWER THE FOLLOWING.

1. The disorders of autism include pervasive developmental disorders, autistic like, autistic, high functioning autistic, Rett disorder, and Asperger's syndrome.

2. Six problem areas experienced by children with learning disorders include reasoning, comprehension, verbal skills, reading, writing, and math.

3. Coping, adaptation, and social skills development are greatly dependent on abstract thinking and the ability to generalize from one situation to another. This leads to inappropriate or ineffective behaviors.

4. Developmental disorders may result from a variety of causes. They may be genetic, related to prenatal or perinatal insult, or acquired as a result of illness, injury, and environmental exposures.

5. The term *cognitive functioning* is more appropriate than *intelligence*, because results on tests such as the Bayley III are poorly correlated with intelligence in adulthood. The younger the child is when the test is administered, the lower the correlation the test result has with adult IQ.

Activity E CONSIDER THE SCENARIO AND ANSWER THE QUESTIONS.

1. It is important to explain that the recent change in his environment and new uncertainty may be causing Kendall's new negative behaviors. Kendall's parents should be taught interventions to help Kendall cope with the current change. Explain that completely eliminating or preventing disruptions or change in the environment is impossible, so it is more productive to help establish ways to deal with the change. For example, allowing Kendall to participate in setting up his new room and placing his toys where he wants them may be helpful. Providing him with pictures of his family and perhaps his old house may also help. Explain that this behavior should improve after Kendall feels more secure in his new environment.

2. Kendall's parents need to be taught home-based and behavioral strategies to deal with their child's temper tantrums and head banging. In some cases, medication administration may be warranted. Referral to a mental health counselor or practitioner may be helpful to develop coping strategies. Kendall's parents should learn to anticipate schedule changes and communicate them to the child. Although difficult, Kendall's parents must reward positive behavior and ignore the negative behavior. They should walk away and ignore Kendall's temper tantrums, yet reward him when he accepts and deals with a new situation.

3. Kendall's parents are going to need different community resources to help them. They will benefit from social support, education, and respite care. Education should be initiated as soon as possible. A support group in the community with other parents, children, and families dealing with autism will be helpful. Allowing Kendall to participate in school and community activities will help him to develop social skills. Respite care will be important for Kendall's parents to give them a break from the intense day-to-day care and attention Kendall needs.

SECTION III: PRACTICING FOR NCLEX

Activity F CHOOSE THE BEST ANSWER.

1. **Answer: d**
   RATIONALE: The presence of excellent language skills suggests Asperger's syndrome. The repetitive behavior pattern with the toys, along with observation of communication and social impairments would suggest autistic disorder. Below-average intellectual function is a sign of mental retardation. Loss of attained skills is a sign of Rett disorder, which occurs only in girls.

2. **Answer: d**
   RATIONALE: Children with learning disorders in one area may have exceptional capabilities in another area. Learning disorders do not predict intelligence. They should not be considered deficits, but, rather, different responses to information. Special education is focused on the area of the learning disorder rather than all areas of the child's education.

3. **Answer: a**
   RATIONALE: Children with mental retardation may display self-stimulating behaviors, such as slapping themselves on the head. Brushing her teeth with supervision and knowing cat and dog sounds are normal for this age. Having trouble with "r," "l," and "y" sounds is not unusual and may continue until age 7.

4. **Answer: c**
   RATIONALE: The nurse will teach the parents about the child's specific difficulty as part of the plan. Encouraging parents to provide a personal space for the child is an intervention meant to promote autonomy and responsibility for a child with delayed growth and development. Regularly checking up on the child is a preventative measure to promote safety for a child with a developmental disorder. Learning facial expressions is important when a child has impaired communication skills.

5. **Answer: c**
   RATIONALE: Upward slanted palpebral fissures are typical physical features associated with Down syndrome. Large ears and a long face are typical of fragile X syndrome. A flat, recessed forehead is typical of brachycephaly.

6. **Answer: b**
   RATIONALE: A child with impaired adaptive functioning may not be able to communicate using language and speech skills. The inability to copy a phone number or sentence, or to read well are learning disorders.

7. **Answer: b**
   RATIONALE: Mentally retarded children are unable to think in abstract terms. Instruction must be given using simple, concrete terms and brief, simple sentences. Being consistent with expectations, individualizing the teaching methods, being patient, and rewarding successes are good teaching techniques for general use.

8. **Answer: d**

   RATIONALE: Chromosomal analysis is performed on a blood sample, so the child would need a topical anesthetic for the sampling site. Many young children are unable to remain still long enough for a CT scan and require a sedative. MRI machines are noisy, so patients may be given headphones to listen to music during the procedure. It is necessary to note the child's diet prior to metabolic screening.

9. **Answer: c**

   RATIONALE: Helping parents interpret test results is one of the roles the nurse performs. Psychologists will perform the Wechsler and Stanford-Binet tests. A trained genetic counselor will provide genetic counseling.

10. **Answer: c**

    RATIONALE: Teaching how to plan schedules and routines would be part of the education plan. Providing education to build social skills, conducting developmental assessments of the child, and linking the family to support groups are all nursing interventions for providing services to the child.

CHAPTER 31

SECTION I: ASSESSING YOUR UNDERSTANDING

Activity A MATCH THE TERM IN COLUMN A WITH THE CORRECT DESCRIPTION IN COLUMN B.

1. c   **2.** a   **3.** d   **4.** b

Activity B FILL IN THE BLANKS.

1. Unknown
2. Chelation
3. Smoke inhalation
4. Atopy

Activity C BRIEFLY ANSWER THE FOLLOWING.

1. Establish a patent *airway*; assist *breathing*; provide *circulatory* support; assess *disability*; *expose* the body; (*Fahrenheit*) provide a heat source; *get* vital signs, *history*, and head-to-toe examination; and *inspect* the patient's back.

2. Raccoon eyes is a sign of basilar skull fracture that places the child at risk for intracranial hemorrhage, respiratory depression, respiratory arrest, and cerebral edema.

3. In a pediatric emergency, the nurse must confirm that a thorough neurologic and cardiovascular examination has been performed before any pain medication is administered.

SECTION II: APPLYING YOUR KNOWLEDGE

Activity D CONSIDER THE FOLLOWING SCENARIO AND ANSWER THE QUESTIONS.

1. The signs and symptoms of croup typically are mild to moderate, with the child not exhibiting the toxic appearance that is usually seen with epiglottitis. Usually, the child with croup has evidence of an upper airway infection that progresses to fever, barking cough, inspiratory stridor, tachycardia, tachypnea, retractions, and altered breath sounds. Crystal's appearance is toxic and her signs and symptoms reflect a rapid onset, as evidenced by her mother's statement that "she was fine a couple of hours ago." In addition, she has a high fever. Fever may or may not be present with croup.

2. Crystal needs to be monitored closely in a controlled medical environment because of the increased risk for airway obstruction. The nurse also should have equipment for emergency intubation and/or tracheostomy readily available. Crystal should be allowed to assume whatever position is comfortable for her. In addition, the nurse should advocate to avoid any invasive or disturbing procedures that may cause agitation and prevent attempts to have the child lay down, because these may lead to laryngospasm, which would completely block her airway. Antibiotic therapy would be initiated to treat the underlying organism. The nurse would provide comfort measures, including measures to reduce Crystal's fever.

SECTION III: PRACTICING FOR NCLEX

Activity E CHOOSE THE BEST ANSWER.

1. a   **2.** c   **3.** a   **4.** d   **5.** b
6. b